Intercollegiate MRCS

Clinical Problem Solving EMQS

Volume 1

Christopher L H Chan BSc (Hons) MB BS FRCS
Consultant General and Colorectal Surgeon
Barts and The London
Queen Mary's School of Medicine and Dentistry
University of London

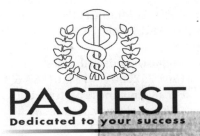

PASTEST
Dedicated to your success

© 2004 PASTEST LTD
Egerton Court
Parkgate Estate
Knutsford
Cheshire WA16 8DX

Telephone: 01565 752000

A percentage of the questions were previously published in *MRCS System Modules: The Complete Test* and *MRCS Core Modules: The Complete Test*.

First edition 2004
ISBN 1 904627 23 4

A catalogue record for this book is available from the British Library.

The information contained within this book was obtained by the author from reliable sources. However, while every effort has been made to ensure its accuracy, no responsibility for loss, damage or injury occasioned to any person acting or refraining from action as a result of information contained herein can be accepted by the publishers or author.

PasTest Revision Books and Intensive Courses
PasTest has been established in the field of postgraduate medical education since 1972, providing revision books and intensive study courses for doctors preparing for their professional examinations.
Books and courses are available for the following specialties:
MRCP Part 1 and Part 2, MRCPCH Part 1 and Part 2, MRCOG, DRCOG, MRCGP, MRCPsych, DCH, FRCA, MRCS and PLAB.
For further details contact:
**PasTest, Freepost, Knutsford, Cheshire WA16 7BR
Tel: 01565 752000   Fax: 01565 650264
E-mail: enquiries@pastest.co.uk
Web site: www.pastest.co.uk**

Typeset by Breeze Limited, Manchester
Printed by Alden Group Limited, Oxfordshire

CONTENTS

PREFACE

This book is primarily intended for candidates sitting the Part 2 (Clinical Problem Solving) section of the Intercollegiate Membership examination of the Surgical Royal Colleges of Great Britain and Ireland (MRCS). The extended matching questions have been specifically structured to reflect the new changes in the syllabus and examination of the Surgical Royal Colleges of Great Britain and Ireland.

The goal of such a book is to help assess knowledge and provide an adjunct to reading, in addition to alerting one to areas that require further study. This book covers many of the 'most popular' topics that appear in the MRCS examination. EMQ practice will increase overall knowledge and detailed explanations have been written to aid revision. The explanations will also be useful to candidates in other parts of the examination.

I hope that this book will not be restricted only to candidates sitting the MRCS examination but will be of use to Final Year medical students.

Christopher L H Chan

CONTRIBUTORS

Editor:

Christopher L H Chan BSc (Hons) MB BS FRCS, Consultant General and Colorectal Surgeon, Barts and the London, Queen Mary's School of Medicine and Dentistry

Contributor:

Stuart Enoch MSSS MRCSEd MRCS (Eng), PhD Research Fellow of the Royal Colleges of Surgeons of Edinburgh and Ireland

EXAMINATION TECHNIQUE

The written section of the new Intercollegiate Membership examination of the Surgical Royal Colleges of Great Britain and Ireland has undergone recent revision (2004) and now comprises two written papers: Part 1 for Applied Basic Sciences (ABS) and Part 2 for Clinical Problem Solving (CPS). The Part 1 ABS paper consists of multiple true false questions only. Candidates are allowed 3 hours for the paper. The Part 2 CPS consists of extended matching questions only and is presently $2\frac{1}{2}$ hours in length but from April 2005 will last 3 hours.

Pacing yourself accurately during the examination to finish on time, or with time to spare, is essential. There are two common mistakes which cause good candidates to fail the MRCS written examinations. These are neglecting to read the directions and questions carefully enough and failing to fill in the computer answer card properly. You must read the instructions given to candidates at the beginning of each section of the paper to ensure that you complete the answer sheet correctly.

You must also decide on a strategy to follow with regard to marking your answer sheet. The answer sheet is read by an automatic document reader and transfers the information to a computer. It is critical that the answer sheet is filled in clearly and accurately using the pencils provided. Failure to fill in your name and your examination correctly could result in the rejection of your paper.

Some candidates mark their answers directly onto the computer sheet as they go through the question, others prefer to make a note of their answers on the question paper, and reserve time at the end to transfer their answers onto the computer sheet. If you choose the first method, there is a chance that you may decide to change your answer after a second reading. If you do change your answer on the computer sheet, you must ensure that your original is thoroughly erased. If you choose the second method, make sure that you allow enough time to transfer your answers methodically onto the computer sheet, as rushing at this stage could introduce some costly mistakes. You will find it less confusing if you transfer your marks after you have completed each section of the examination. You must ensure that you have left sufficient time to transfer your marks from the question paper to the answer sheet. You should also be aware that no additional time will be given at the end of the examination to allow you to transfer your marks.

If you find that you have time left at the end of the examination, there can be a temptation to re-read your answers time and time again, so that even those that seemed straightforward will start to look less convincing. In this situation, first thoughts are usually best, don't alter your initial answers unless you are sure.

You must also ensure that you read the question (both stem and items) carefully. Regard each item as being independent of every other item, each referring to a specific quantum of knowledge. For the CPS section, it is important to choose the *most likely* answer as there may be more than one 'correct' answer. For every correct answer you will gain a mark (+1). Marks will not be deducted for a wrong answer. Equally, you will not gain a mark if you mark both true and false.

For this reason you should answer every question as you have nothing to lose. If you do not know the answer to a question, you should make an educated guess – you may well get the answer right and gain a mark.

If you feel that you need to spend more time puzzling over a question, leave it and, if you have time, return to it. Make sure you have collected all the marks you can before you come back to any difficult questions.

Multiple choice questions are not designed to trick you or confuse you, they are designed to test your knowledge of medicine. Accept each question at face value.

The aim of this book is to give you practice and therefore aid revision for the Part 2 CPS paper. The broad range of questions is to test your knowledge on specific subjects.

Working through the questions in this book will help you to identify your weak subject areas. In the last few weeks before the exam it will be important for you to avoid minor unimportant areas and concentrate on the most important subject areas covered in the exam.

ABBREVIATIONS

AAA	abdominal aortic aneurysm
ABPI	arterial blood pressure index
ACE	angiotensin-converting enzyme
ACTH	adrenocorticotropic hormone
ADH	antidiuretic hormone
α-FP	alpha-fetoprotein
AIDS	acquired immunodeficiency syndrome
ASD	atrial septal defect
AXR	abdominal X-ray
BP	blood pressure
C1 etc. segment	cervical spinal segment
CBD	common bile duct
CEA	carcinoembryonic antigen
CIN	cervical intraepithelial neoplasia
CMF	cyclophosphamide, methotrexate and 5-FU (regimen)
CNS	central nervous system
COPD	chronic obstructive pulmonary disease
CRP	C-reactive protein
CSF	cerebrospinal fluid
CT	computed tomography
CVA	cerebral vascular accident
CXR	chest X-ray
DMSA	dimercaptosuccinic acid
DTPA	diethylene triamine pentacetic acid
DVT	deep venous thrombosis
ECG	electrocardiogram
ERCP	endoscopic retrograde cholangiopancreatography
ESR	erythrocyte sedimentation ratio
ESWL	extracorporeal shock wave lithotripsy
EUA	examination under anaesthesia
FAP	familial adenomatous polyposis
FBC	full blood count
GCS	Glasgow coma scale
GI	gastrointestinal
GP	general practitioner
β-hCG	human chorionic gonadotrophin
HIV	human immunodeficiency virus
HLA	human leukocyte antigen
IV	intravenous

IVU	intravenous urogram
JVP	jugular venous pressure
KUB	kidney and upper bladder
MEN	multiple endocrine neoplasia
MI	myocardial infarction
MRA	magnetic resonance angiography
MRI	magnetic resonance imaging
MRSA	methicillin-resistant *Staphylococcus aureus*
MSU	mid-stream urine specimen
NEC	necrotising enterocolitis
NSAID	non-specific anti-inflammatory drug
PCNL	percutaneous nephrolithotomy
P_{CO_2}	partial pressure of carbon dioxide
PDS	polydioxanone
PE	pulmonary embolism
P_{O_2}	partial pressure of oxygen
PP	pulse pressure
PSA	prostatic specific antigen
PTFE	polytetrafluoroethylene
PUJ	pelvi-ureteric junction
RTA	road traffic accident
RUQ	right upper quadrant
SCC	squamous-cell carcinoma
SFA	superficial femoral artery
SLR	straight leg raise
SMA	superior mesenteric artery
T1 etc. segment	thoracic spinal segment
TB	tuberculosis
TEDS	thromboembolic deterrent stockings
TIA	transient ischaemic attack
TPA	tissue plasminogen activator
TURBT	transurethral resection of bladder tumour
TURP	transurethral resection of the prostate
UTI	urinary tract infection
VIP	vasoactive intestinal peptide
VSD	ventricular septal defect
WBC	white blood cells
WCC	white cell count

QUESTIONS

QUESTIONS

1 THEME: CONSENT FOR SURGICAL TREATMENT

A Apply to make the child a ward of court
B No, surgery cannot proceed
C Obtain consent from patient
D Obtain consent from wife
E Yes, surgery can proceed

For each of the following situations, select the most likely answer from the above list. Each option may be used once, more than once, or not at all.

☐ **1** A 24-year-old man found unconscious by the roadside is brought to hospital by ambulance. It is evident that the patient's condition is rapidly deteriorating because of an expanding extradural haematoma and he is unable to give consent. His wife had been contacted and is at the hospital but has expressed her refusal to allow him to be operated on. Would you proceed against her wishes?

☐ **2** A member of an extreme religious sect has brought their 11-year-old son to hospital with generalised peritonitis from a perforated appendix. The child's condition deteriorates and he needs a laparotomy which both parents adamantly refuse, saying that he will recover through the fervent prayers of members of the sect. Despite repeated attempts by the surgical team to persuade the parents of this child, they refuse to give consent for the surgical treatment that the surgeon deems to be essential. What option is available to the surgeon?

☐ **3** A 70-year-old woman with severe psychiatric illness is undergoing compulsory psychiatric treatment, having been sectioned under the Mental Health Act. She has a fall in the psychiatry unit and sustains a fracture of the neck of the right femur for which she is referred for surgical treatment The orthopaedic surgeon thinks that internal fixation of the fracture is the best management, in agreement with her psychiatrist. Her psychiatric state does not allow her to give informed consent for surgery. What process should follow?

☐ **4** A 63-year-old man with a brain tumour refuses any surgery and expresses his wish formally in writing. He is judged to be mentally competent. The following day he enters into a coma and his wife, who was abroad, arrives at his bedside and demands that surgical treatment is commenced. Can surgery proceed?

2 THEME: DEATH AND THE LAW

A   Any medical practitioner
B   Coroner
C   Coroner's officer
D   Medical practitioner who attended during previous 14 days
E   Registrar of births and deaths

For each of the statements below, select the most likely answer from the above list. Each option may be used once, more than once, or not at all.

☐ **1**   Certify death.

☐ **2**   Issue immediate death certificate.

☐ **3**   Call an inquest.

☐ **4**   Send information concerning the cause of death to the Office of Population Censuses and Surveys.

3 THEME: DEATH CERTIFICATES

A   Ask families for permission for a postmortem
B   Ask the GP to issue a death certificate
C   Issue a death certificate
D   Order a hospital postmortem
E   Report to the coroner

For each of the situations below, select the most likely answer from the above list. Each option may be used once, more than once, or not at all.

☐ **1**   A 20-year-old man was found emaciated in a derelict building. On examination he had two liver abscesses and was human immuno-deficiency virus (HIV) positive, and died 5 days after admission to hospital.

☐ **2**   A 50-year-old man was admitted with jaundice secondary to cholangiocarcinoma. His tumour was resected, but the patient died 5 days later from a myocardial infarction (MI).

4 THEME: CANCER THERAPY OPTIONS

A Hormonal manipulation
B Radiotherapy and steroids
C Surgical resection
D Systemic chemotherapy

For each of the clinical scenarios listed below, select the most appropriate management options from the above list. Each option may be used once, more than once, or not at all.

☐ **1** Recurrent non-Hodgkin's lymphoma

☐ **2** Isolated pulmonary metastasis from colorectal cancer

☐ **3** Residual anal squamous cell carcinoma (SCC) after local radiotherapy

☐ **4** Metastatic prostatic carcinoma not involving bone

☐ **5** Diffuse intracranial metastatic melanoma

5 THEME: MALIGNANT MELANOMA

A Acral lentiginous melanoma
B Amelanotic melanoma
C Lentigo maligna melanoma
D Nodular melanoma
E Superficial spreading melanoma

For each of the scenarios given below, select the correct type of cutaneous malignant melanoma from the above list. Each option may be used once, more than once, or not at all.

☐ **1** Occurs within a Hutchinson's melanotic freckle.

☐ **2** Has a predilection for sites with thick epidermis such as the sole(s) of the feet.

☐ **3** Usually occurs on the face of elderly patients.

☐ **4** Is the commonest type of cutaneous malignant melanoma.

6   THEME: HISTOLOGICAL TUMOUR TYPES

A   Hamartoma
B   Neoplastic polyp
C   Neuroendocrine tumour
D   Gastrointestinal stromal tumour

For each of the tumours/polyps listed below, select the correct histological type they belong to from the above list. Each option may be used once, more than once, or not at all.

☐ **1** Villous adenoma

☐ **2** Peutz–Jeghers polyp

☐ **3** Juvenile polyp

☐ **4** Carcinoid tumour

☐ **5** Insulinoma

☐ **6** Leiomyosarcoma   — CD 117

☐ **7** Glucagonoma

7   THEME: TUMOUR MARKERS

A   Acid phosphatase
B   α-fetoprotein
C   β-hCG
D   Carcinoembryonic antigen (CEA)
E   Paraproteins

For each of the tumours listed below, select the most appropriate serum marker from the above list. Each option may be used once, more than once, or not at all.

☐ **1** Choriocarcinoma

☐ **2** Hepatoma

☐ **3** Prostatic carcinoma

☐ **4** Colorectal cancer

☐ **5** Multiple myeloma

8   THEME: CHEMOTHERAPY REGIMENS

A   Breast carcinoma
B   Colorectal carcinoma
C   Malignant carcinoid
D   Testicular seminoma

For each of the tumour scenarios listed below, select the most appropriate chemotherapeutic regimen from the above list. Each option may be used once, more than once, or not at all.

☐ **1** Combination of 5-fluorouracil and folinic acid.

☐ **2** Combination of cyclophosphamide, methotrexate and 5-fluorouracil.

☐ **3** Combination of bleomycin, cisplatin and etoposide.

9 THEME: TESTICULAR TUMOURS

A Choriocarcinoma
B Seminoma
C Teratoma

For each of the statements below, select the most likely testicular tumour type from the above list. Each option may be used once, more than once, or not at all.

☐ **1** Secrete α-fetoprotein (α-FP) in approximately 70% of cases.

☐ **2** Secrete β-hCG in less than 10% of cases.

☐ **3** Secrete either α-FP or β-hCG in about 90% of cases.

☐ **4** Secrete β-hCG in approximately 60% of cases.

☐ **5** Almost always secrete β-hCG.

10 THEME: HORMONE-SECRETING TUMOURS

A ACTH
B α-Fetoprotein
C Calcitonin
D Erythropoietin
E Growth hormone
F 5-Hydroxytryptamine

For each of the tumours listed below, select the most likely hormone produced by the tumour from the above list. Each option may be used once, more than once, or not at all.

☐ **1** Testicular teratoma

☐ **2** Bronchial carcinoma

☐ **3** Medullary thyroid carcinoma

☐ **4** Carcinoid tumour

☐ **5** Hypernephroma

11 THEME: SKIN LESIONS

A   Central keratin plug
B   Intraepidermal (in situ) squamous carcinoma
C   Intraepithelial adenocarcinoma
D   Keratin pearl formation
E   Palisading basal cells at the periphery of tumour islands
F   S-100 positive on immunohistochemical staining

For each of the lesions listed below, select the most appropriate characteristics from the above list. Each option may be used once, more than once, or not at all.

☐ **1** Malignant melanoma

☐ **2** Basal cell carcinoma

☐ **3** Squamous cell carcinoma

☐ **4** Bowen's disease

☐ **5** Keratoacanthoma

12 THEME: LOCAL ANAESTHETIC AGENTS

A   Amethocaine   E   Dibucaine
B   Bupivacaine   F   Prilocaine
C   Cinchocaine   G   None of above
D   Cocaine

For each scenario listed below, select the most appropriate local anaesthetic agent from the list of options above. Each option may be used once, more than once, or not at all.

☐ **1** This agent is commonly used for conjunctival anaesthesia.

☐ **2** This agent has previously caused deaths when used in Bier's blocks.

☐ **3** This agent causes sympathetic stimulation.

13 THEME: OPERATIVE MANAGEMENT

A   Cancel surgery
B   Carry on with surgery regardless
C   Conservative management
D   Immediate surgery and intensive care unit booking
E   Wait 4 weeks
F   Wait 6 months

For each of the clinical scenarios described below, select the most appropriate management plan from the above list. Each option may be used once, more than once, or not at all.

☐ **1** A 25-year-old woman is diagnosed with acute appendicitis at the beginning of the third trimester of her pregnancy.

☐ **2** A 25-year-old woman is diagnosed with acute appendicitis and is taking the oral contraceptive pill.

☐ **3** A 30-year-old woman is on your waiting list for a right inguinal hernia repair but is on the oral contraceptive pill.

14 THEME: TUMOUR TYPE

A   Adenocarcinoma   D   Sarcoma
B   Lymphoma   E   Squamous cell carcinoma
C   Melanoma

Which of the above histological tumour types most clearly fits the clinical picture below? Each option may be used once, more than once, or not at all.

☐ **1** Tumour arising in association with the Epstein–Barr virus.

☐ **2** Tumour arising within the quadriceps muscle.

☐ **3** Tumour arising in association with human papillomavirus types 16 and 18.

☐ **4** Tumour arising in Barrett's oesophagus.

☐ **5** Krukenberg tumour.

15 THEME: PARANEOPLASTIC SYNDROMES

A	Colon carcinoma	D	Pancreatic carcinoma
B	Lymphoma	E	Renal carcinoma
C	Multiple myeloma	F	Thymoma

For each of the clinical systemic manifestations below, select the tumour most likely to produce these effects from the above list. Each option may be used once, more than once, or not at all.

☐ **1** Myasthenia gravis

☐ **2** Polycythaemia

☐ **3** Hypercalcaemia

☐ **4** Hyperglycaemia

16 THEME: MODE OF TUMOUR SPREAD

A   Blood-borne spread
B   Local invasion
C   Lymphatic spread
D   Transcoelomic spread

For each of the tumours below, select the predominant mode of spread from the above list. Each option may be used once, more than once, or not at all.

☐ **1** Seminoma of the testis

☐ **2** Cutaneous basal cell carcinoma

☐ **3** Papillary thyroid carcinoma

☐ **4** Follicular thyroid carcinoma

☐ **5** Ovarian carcinoma

17 THEME: ARTERIAL BLOOD GAS ANALYSIS/ACID–BASE BALANCE

A   Compensated respiratory alkalosis
B   Metabolic acidosis
C   Metabolic alkalosis
D   Respiratory acidosis
E   Respiratory alkalosis

From the options above, select the most appropriate description of acid–base status from the list below. Each option may be used once, more than once, or not at all.

☐ **1**   A 64-year-old man arrives collapsed at the Emergency Department with a suspected leaking abdominal aortic aneurysm. Blood gases show: pH 7.05, P_{CO_2} 3.5 kPa, P_{O_2} 12 kPa and bicarbonate concentration 7 mmol/l.

☐ **2**   A 72-year-old man becomes confused on the ward 6 hours after major abdominal surgery. Blood gases show: pH 7.24, P_{CO_2} 8 kPa, P_{O_2} 8 kPa and bicarbonate concentration 25 mmol/l.

☐ **3**   A 70-year-old man with a 3-week history of vomiting has a blood gas picture demonstrating: pH 7.56, P_{CO_2} 7.2 kPa, P_{O_2} 13 kPa and bicarbonate concentration 45 mmol/l.

18 THEME: SHOCK

A   Cardiogenic shock
B   Fat embolism
C   Hypovolaemic shock
D   Thromboembolism

For each of the scenarios listed below, select the most likely diagnosis from the above list. Each option may be used once, more than once, or not at all.

☐ **1** A 26-year-old man with a comminuted closed fracture of the femur shaft undergoes intramedullary nail fixation. Two days post-operatively, he develops a pyrexia, shortness of breath and a tachycardia.

☐ **2** A 72-year-old man with an underlying prostate carcinoma sustains a femoral shaft fracture. He undergoes intramedullary nail fixation. At post-operative day 7, he develops shortness of breath, hypotension and a tachycardia.

☐ **3** A 60-year-old man develops sudden back pain and is brought to the Emergency Department with a swollen, tense abdomen. He is tachycardic, with a low-volume pulse and low BP.

19 THEME: 5-YEAR SURVIVAL RATES OF TUMOURS

A	< 5%	E	50–60%
B	25%	F	70–75%
C	> 95%	G	90–95%
D	5–10%		

For each of the clinical scenarios listed below, select the most likely 5-year survival rate from the above list. Each option may be used once, more than once, or not at all.

☐ **1** Carcinoid of the appendix

☐ **2** Duke's A rectal cancer

☐ **3** Oesophageal cancer

☐ **4** Pancreatic carcinoma

☐ **5** Metastatic prostatic cancer

☐ **6** Duke's B rectal cancer

20 THEME: LYMPH NODES

A	Deep inguinal	D	Superficial inguinal
B	External iliac	E	Supraclavicular
C	Para-aortic		

For each of the conditions listed below, choose the area in which lymphadenopathy would be most likely to occur. Each option may be used once, more than once, or not at all.

☐ **1** A 20-year-old man with testicular teratoma.

☐ **2** A 40-year-old woman with cervical cancer.

☐ **3** A young man with a perianal abscess.

☐ **4** An 80-year-old man with rectal carcinoma.

21 THEME: TYPES OF ULCERATION

A	Curling's ulcer	D	Neuropathic ulcers
B	Cushing's ulcer	E	Pyoderma gangrenosum
C	Marjolin's ulcer		

For each of the clinical scenarios listed below, select the lesion most likely to occur in that scenario from the above list. Each option may be used once, more than once, or not at all.

☐ **1** Squamous cell carcinoma in a chronic venous ulcer.

☐ **2** Head injury.

☐ **3** Major burns.

☐ **4** Inflammatory bowel disease.

Questions

22 THEME: PATHOLOGIES OF THE FEMORO-INGUINAL REGION

A	Psoas abscess	G	Local abscess
B	Obturator hernia	H	Strangulated inguinal hernia
C	Femoral aneurysm	I	Infected sebaceous cyst
D	Strangulated femoral hernia	J	Saphena varix
E	Enlargement of psoas bursa		
F	False aneurysm of the femoral artery		

For each of the clinical scenarios listed below, select the lesion most likely to occur in that scenario from the above list. Each option may be used once, more than once, or not at all.

☐ **1** A 60-year-old lady presents to the A&E with a temperature of 37.6°C and vomiting of 48 hours duration. On examination, a localised swelling below and lateral to the right pubic tubercle is noticed. The swelling is tender and irreducible with no cough impulse.

☐ **2** A 46-year-old lady presents with a soft, non-tender swelling over the medial side of her right thigh below and lateral to the pubic tubercle. The swelling has got a bluish tinge and disappears on lying down. She is well systemically but has got bilateral varicose veins.

☐ **3** A 35-year-old man of Asian origin presents with a painless, fluctuant swelling over the upper medial side of his left thigh. He has been previously treated for tuberculosis. His ESR is 113. He has also got some tenderness over the lower spine and X-ray reveals some opacity in this region.

☐ **4** A 28-year-old IV drug abuser presents with a mildly tender, pulsatile swelling over his right femoral triangle. He gives a history of considerable bleeding from the wound before the swelling developed. He is apyrexial and systemically well.

23 THEME: ABDOMINAL DISEASE

A	Appendix mass	E	Intussusception
B	Caecal carcinoma	F	Meckel's diverticulum
C	Coeliac disease	G	Mesenteric ischaemia
D	Crohn's disease		

For each of the patients below, select the most likely diagnosis from the above list. Each option may be used once, more than once, or not at all.

☐ 1 An 80-year-old lady with atrial fibrillation has a 4-day history of abdominal pain and some rectal bleeding.

☐ 2 A 16-year-old boy presents with a 6-month history of diarrhoea, vomiting and vague right iliac fossa mass. He has a microcytic anaemia.

☐ 3 An 18-year-old girl presents with a 4-day history of pain in the right iliac fossa, a temperature of 38 °C and diarrhoea.

24 THEME: INVESTIGATIONS FOR ABDOMINAL PAIN

A	CT abdomen	E	Mesenteric angiography
B	ECG	F	Supine abdominal X-ray
C	Erect chest X-ray	G	Urea
D	FBC		

For each of the patients below, select the most likely specific diagnostic investigation from the above list. Each option may be used once, more than once, or not at all.

☐ 1 An 18-year-old man presents with 24 hours of generalised abdominal pain, which has now shifted to the right iliac fossa.

☐ 2 A 59-year-old woman with a history of rheumatoid arthritis treated with NSAIDs, gold and steroids, presents with 4 hours of acute abdominal pain. This was made worse by the ambulance ride.

☐ 3 An 85-year-old woman presents with profuse, fresh, red rectal bleeding. She is hypotensive, with a fast irregular pulse.

☐ 4 A 62-year-old woman is admitted with vomiting, colicky abdominal pain and a distended abdomen. She has previously undergone multiple gynaecological operations.

25 THEME: ABDOMINAL PAIN INVESTIGATIONS – DIAGNOSTIC

A   Abdominal ultrasound
B   Angiography (mesenteric)
C   Barium enema
D   Barium meal – small bowel follow-through
E   CT
F   Erect chest X-ray
G   FBC
H   Serum amylase
I   Supine abdominal X-ray

For each of the patients described below, select the most likely investigation from the list of options above. Each option may be used once, more than once, or not at all.

☐ **1**   A 70-year-old man is admitted with severe central and epigastric pain and vomiting. On examination he has bruising on his flanks.

☐ **2**   An 18-year-old man has a 2-year history of central abdominal pain, which now has moved to the right iliac fossa. He has had two episodes of loose stools over the past 6 months.

☐ **3**   A middle-aged woman presents with epigastric pain. She has shallow breathing, tachycardia, but is normotensive. She has rheumatoid arthritis and receives regular gold injections and takes oral steroids and diclofenac. She has taken an increased steroid dose over the past week because of a chest infection.

☐ **4**   An elderly woman presents with a history of copious rectal bleeding over a 7-hour period. She is tachycardic and hypotensive.

26 THEME: INVESTIGATIONS OF THE GASTROINTESTINAL TRACT

A Colonoscopy
B CT scan
C Fully prepared barium enema
D Proctoscopy
E Small bowel follow-through

For each of the patients described below, select the most likely investigation from the list of options above. Each option may be used once, more than once, or not at all.

☐ **1** A 60-year-old man had banding of haemorrhoids 8 weeks previously and continues to pass dark blood and mucus per rectum.

☐ **2** A 50-year-old woman with psychiatric problems presents with abdominal distension and absolute constipation.

27 THEME: PANCREATITIS

A Acute pancreatitis
B Acute-on-chronic pancreatitis
C Biliary obstruction
D Cancer of the head of the pancreas
E Pancreatic pseudocyst

For each of the patients described below, select the most likely diagnosis from the list of options above. Each option may be used once, more than once, or not at all.

☐ **1** A 43-year-old man, with a history of alcohol abuse, presents with pain radiating to his back, which is relieved by leaning forward. He has obstructive jaundice and has recent weight loss.

☐ **2** A 52-year-old man who drinks 14 units/day and is a heavy smoker presents with acute onset of epigastric pain. He has a history of chronic pancreatitis, steatorrhoea and also has a palpable abdominal mass.

☐ **3** A 40-year-old man with a history of sudden onset abdominal pain and vomiting has an increased serum amylase. He has no previous history of pancreatitis.

28 THEME: CHOLECYSTECTOMY

A   Cholestyramine
B   Elective cholecystectomy
C   Emergency cholecystectomy
D   Endoscopic retrograde cholangiopancreatography (ERCP)
E   Lithotripsy

For each of the patients described below, select the most likely treatment from the list of options above. Each option may be used once, more than once, or not at all.

☐ **1** A 77-year-old woman presents with abdominal pain and jaundice. Ultrasound reveals stones in the common bile duct. She is unwell and not fit for theatre.

☐ **2** A young woman presents to the outpatient department with a history of fat intolerance and abdominal pain in the right upper quadrant. An ultrasound scan reveals that she has gallstones. Upper GI endoscopy was normal.

29 THEME: PANCREATIC TUMOUR

A   Dumping syndrome
B   Glucagonoma
C   Insulinoma
D   VIPoma
E   Zollinger–Ellison syndrome

For each of the patients described below, select the most likely pancreatic tumour from the list of options above. Each option may be used once, more than once, or not at all.

☐ **1** A vicar who missed breakfast swore during his sermon, but felt better after a late breakfast.

☐ **2** A 52-year-old man with hypercalcaemia suffers from recurrent gastric ulcers.

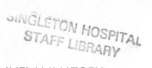
30 THEME: SIDE-EFFECTS OF TREATMENT FOR INFLAMMATORY
    BOWEL DISEASE

A	Azathioprine	D	Metronidazole
B	Corticosteroids	E	Sulfasalazine
C	Methotrexate		

For each of the options listed below, select the most likely associated side-effects from the list of drugs above. Each option may be used once, more than once, or not at all.

☐ **1** Irreversible peripheral neuropathy

☐ **2** Reversible infertility due to oligospermia

☐ **3** Osteoporosis

☐ **4** Cataracts

☐ **5** Hepatic fibrosis

☐ **6** Pneumonitis

31 THEME: SURGICAL INVESTIGATIONS

A	Abdominal and pelvic CT scan	E	Colonoscopy
B	Abdominal ultrasound	F	ERCP
C	Barium enema	G	Gastrografin enema
D	Capsule endoscopy	H	Small bowel follow-through

For each of the conditions listed below, select the most appropriate investigation from the above list. Each option may be used once, more than once, or not at all.

☐ **1** A suspected, acutely obstructing large bowel cancer.

☐ **2** Empyema of the gallbladder.

☐ **3** Colonic diverticular abscess.

☐ **4** Terminal ileal Crohn's disease.

☐ **5** Colonic anastomotic leak (day 4) post-operatively.

32 THEME: SURGICAL INVESTIGATIONS

A	Abdominal CT scan	F	Gastrografin enema
B	Abdominal ultrasound	G	Small bowel follow-through
C	Barium enema (double contrast)	H	Capsule endoscopy
D	Colonoscopy		
E	Endoscopic retrograde cholangio-pancreatography (ERCP)		

For each of the following scenarios, select the most appropriate investigation from the above list. Each option may be used once, more than once, or not at all.

☐ **1** Psoas abscess.

☐ **2** Small bowel tumour.

☐ **3** Colovesical fistula.

☐ **4** Pancreatic necrosis.

33 THEME: ABDOMINAL DISEASE

A	Crohn's disease	D	Peutz–Jeghers syndrome
B	Diverticular disease	E	Ulcerative colitis
C	Familial adenomatous polyposis		

For each of the following conditions below, select the most likely associated disease from the above list. Each option may be used once, more than once, or not at all.

☐ **1** Intra-abdominal desmoids

☐ **2** Ankylosing spondylitis

☐ **3** Enteroenteric fistulas

☐ **4** Perianal sepsis

☐ **5** Pyoderma gangrenosum

☐ **6** Colovesical fistula

34   THEME: HERNIAS

A	Diaphragmatic hernia	E	Obturator hernia
B	Epigastric hernia	F	Perineal hernia
C	Gluteal hernia	G	Sciatic hernia
D	Lumbar hernia	H	Spigelian hernia

For each site of herniation below, select the most likely hernial type from the above list. Each answer may be used once, more than once, or not at all.

☐ **1** Triangle of Petit

☐ **2** Greater sciatic notch

☐ **3** Pelvic floor

☐ **4** Linea semilunaris

35   THEME: POLYPS

A	Inflammatory polyps
B	Metaplastic polyps
C	Peutz–Jeghers polyps
D	Tubular adenomatous polyps
E	Villous adenomatous polyps

For each of the descriptions below, select the most appropriate polyp from the above list. Each option may be used once, more than once, or not at all.

☐ **1** Are usually a consequence of a severe episode of ulcerative colitis.

☐ **2** Are hamartomas.

☐ **3** May cause hypokalaemia.

☐ **4** Have the greatest malignant potential of all colonic polyps.

☐ **5** Are the commonest type of polyp seen in familial adenomatous polyposis.

36 THEME: GASTROINTESTINAL HAEMORRHAGE

A   Colonoscopy
B   CT colonography
C   Double-contrast barium enema
D   Laparoscopy
E   Oesophagogastroduodenoscopy
F   Red cell scan
G   Selective mesenteric angiography
H   Single-contrast enema (gastrografin)

For each of the patients described below, select the most appropriate investigation from the above list. Each option may be used once, more than once, or not at all.

☐ **1** A 45-year-old man is admitted to the Emergency Department with passage of large clots of fresh blood per rectum. There is no evidence of melaena. He is hypotensive, blood pressure 85/40 mmHg and pulse rate 140/min. There is no history of haematemesis, but he is a smoker and drinks 20 units of alcohol per week.

☐ **2** An 85-year-old man is admitted with passage of dark clots per rectum. His blood pressure is 110/70 mmHg and his pulse rate is 90/min. He has recently been complaining of left-sided abdominal pain and a change in bowel habit.

☐ **3** A 25-year-old man attends the outpatient department with three episodes of bright-red rectal bleeding. Rigid sigmoidoscopy and proctoscopy failed to reveal any local causes for the bleeding.

37 THEME: HERNIAS

A Littré's hernia	D Richter's hernia
B Maydl's hernia	E Sliding hernia
C Pantaloon hernia	

For each description listed below, select the most appropriate hernia from the above list. Each option may be used once, more than once, or not at all.

☐ **1** Dual sacs straddling the inferior epigastric vessels.

☐ **2** Two separate loops of bowel.

☐ **3** The posterior wall of the hernial sac is formed by a herniating viscus.

☐ **4** Portion of circumference of the bowel.

☐ **5** Meckel's diverticulum.

38 THEME: JAUNDICE

A Acute cholangitis	E Gilbert's disease
B Biliary colic	F Hepatitis C
C Chronic pancreatitis	G Hepatocellular carcinoma
D Duodenal carcinoma	

For each description listed below, select the most appropriate diagnosis from the above list. Each option may be used once, more than once, or not at all.

☐ **1** A 30-year-old man underwent total colectomy 9 months ago for familial adenomatous polyposis (FAP) and now presents with abdominal pain and jaundice; he is passing dark urine and pale stools.

☐ **2** A 70-year-old man presents with epigastric pain, jaundice, rigors and fever.

☐ **3** A 40-year-old woman presents with right upper quadrant pain. She is nauseated, but does not have jaundice or rigors.

39 THEME: JAUNDICE

A   Cholangiocarcinoma
B   Common bile-duct stone
C   Empyema of the gallbladder
D   Gallbladder calculi
E   Mucocele of the gallbladder

For each of the patients described below, select the most likely diagnosis from the list of options above. Each option may be used once, more than once, or not at all.

☐ 1   A 34-year-old woman presents with a palpable right upper quadrant mass. She has a fever and is generally unwell.

☐ 2   A 30-year-old woman who had an open cholecystectomy presents with obstructive jaundice 48 hours after surgery.

☐ 3   A 38-year-old obese woman presents with right upper quadrant pain. Ultrasound scanning shows a stone in Hartmann's pouch.

40 THEME: PANCREATIC TUMOURS

A   Adenocarcinoma
B   Glucagonoma
C   Insulinoma
D   Non-secreting, islet-cell tumour
E   Zollinger–Ellison syndrome

For each of the patients described below, select the most likely diagnosis from the list of options above. Each option may be used once, more than once, or not at all.

☐ 1   A patient with glossitis and stomatitis has diabetes and a rash on his buttocks.

☐ 2   A patient 4 weeks after parathyroidectomy presents with loss of consciousness and dizziness.

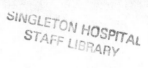

41 THEME: JAUNDICE

A   Hepatic jaundice
B   Post-hepatic jaundice
C   Pre-hepatic jaundice

For each of the clinical findings given below, select the correct type of jaundice from the above list. Each option may be used once, more than once, or not at all.

☐ **1** Bilirubin in the urine.

☐ **2** History of recent foreign travel.

☐ **3** Positive Courvoisier's sign.

☐ **4** Associated pancreatitis.

42 THEME: RECTAL BLEEDING

A   Crohn's disease
B   Familial adenomatous polyposis
C   Fissure in ano
D   Intussusception
E   Meckel's diverticulum
F   Mid-gut volvulus
G   Necrotising enterocolitis
H   Solitary juvenile polyp

For each of the clinical scenarios below, select the most likely cause of rectal bleeding from the above list. Each option may be used once, more than once, or not at all.

☐ **1** A 7-year-old girl presents with weight loss and anaemia.

☐ **2** A 13-year-old boy presents with lower abdominal pain and shock.

☐ **3** A 3-year-old boy presents with painless bleeding, mixed with stool.

☐ **4** A 16-year-old girl presents with painless bleeding, mixed with stool; her father died of colorectal cancer at the age of 35 years.

☐ **5** A 10-month-old girl with a previous history of intermittent bile-stained vomiting has collapsed.

43 THEME: ABDOMINAL PAIN

A   Leaking abdominal aortic aneurysm
B   Pelviureteric obstruction
C   Renal adenocarcinoma
D   Ureteric colic

For each of the statements below, select the most likely diagnosis from the above list. Each option may be used once, more than once, or not at all.

☐ **1**   A 45-year-old man presents with haematuria, loin pain and a loin mass.

☐ **2**   A 22-year-old man experiences loin pain mainly in the morning after drinking four cups of coffee.

☐ **3**   A 70-year-old man presents with loin pain, a pulse rate of 120/min and a BP of 80/60 mmHg.

44 THEME: LOIN PAIN

A   Aortic aneurysm
B   Pancreatitis
C   Pelviureteric junction (PUJ) obstruction
D   Pyelonephritis
E   Renal cell carcinoma
F   Urinary bladder obstruction
G   Urinary calculi

For each of the patients described below, select the most likely diagnosis from the list of options above. Each option may be used once, more than once, or not at all.

☐ **1**   A 30-year-old man presents with loin pain, pyrexia and tachycardia.

☐ **2**   An 18-year-old man presents with pain in his right iliac fossa and microscopic haematuria.

☐ **3**   A woman known to have a previous history of bilateral reflux presents with dysuria, fever and feeling generally unwell.

45 THEME: SCROTAL SWELLINGS

A   Encysted hydrocele of cord
B   Epididymo-orchitis
C   Hydrocele
D   Inguinoscrotal hernia
E   Testicular tumour
F   Torsion of hydatid of Morgagni
G   Varicocele

For each of the patients described below, select the most likely diagnosis from the list of options above. Each option may be used once, more than once, or not at all.

☐ **1** A 42-year-old man presents with a left-sided scrotal swelling. You are unable to get above the swelling, it is compressible, increases on standing, but does not have a positive cough impulse.

☐ **2** An 18-year-old man presents with a sudden onset of testicular pain. On examination you note a firm irregular testis at the apex of the scrotum.

☐ **3** A 22-year-old patient presents with a scrotal swelling that you are unable to get above, it is compressible, increases on standing and has a cough impulse present.

☐ **4** A patient presents with a painless long-standing scrotal swelling which transilluminates. The swelling is not separate from the testis.

46 THEME: JAUNDICE

A Hepatic jaundice
B Post-hepatic jaundice
C Pre-hepatic jaundice

Select the most likely type of jaundice from the above list that would be indicated by the clinical findings or associated with the conditions listed below. Each option may be used once, more than once, or not at all.

☐ **1** Pruritus

☐ **2** Intake of hepatotoxic drugs

☐ **3** Incompatible blood transfusion

☐ **4** Chlorpromazine-induced jaundice

☐ **5** Chronic active hepatitis

☐ **6** Halothane-induced jaundice

☐ **7** Thalassaemia

☐ **8** Sclerosing cholangitis

☐ **9** Hepatic abscesses

☐ **10** Rotor's syndrome

47 THEME: COLORECTAL SURGERY

A	Abdominoperineal resection
B	Anterior resection
C	Hartmann's procedure
D	Ileocolonic bypass
E	Left hemicolectomy
F	Panproctocolectomy
G	Sigmoid colectomy and primary anastomosis
H	Subtotal colectomy
I	Transverse loop colostomy

For each of the patients described below, select the most appropriate surgical option from the above list. Each option may be used once, more than once, or not at all.

☐ **1** A 55-year-old man reattends the surgical outpatient department with rectal bleeding. He has recently completed a course of chemoradiotherapy for a squamous anal carcinoma. He underwent an examination under anaesthesia (EUA) which revealed some residual tumour.

☐ **2** A 30-year-old woman with known ulcerative colitis is admitted as an emergency with abdominal distension, vomiting, rectal bleeding and dehydration. She undergoes a course of conservative medical management but does not respond to steroids and immunosuppressive therapy. Her albumin level is 20 g/l, WBC 25×10^9/l and her colonic diameter on abdominal X-ray is 9 cm.

☐ **3** A 45-year-old man is admitted as an emergency to the Emergency Department with generalised peritonitis. Following aggressive resuscitation he is taken to the operating theatre where a hard 4-cm mass is found in the sigmoid colon. There is gross faecal contamination of the peritoneal cavity. His liver has one umbilicated nodule in the left lobe. The rest of the laparotomy is normal.

48 THEME: MEDIASTINAL CONDITIONS

A   Achalasia
B   Aortic dissection
C   Carcinoma of the oesophagus
D   Mallory–Weiss tear
E   Marfan's syndrome

For each of the scenarios described below, select the most likely diagnosis from the above list. Each option may be used once, more than once, or not at all.

☐ **1** A tall, middle-aged woman presents complaining of a sudden onset of chest pain.

☐ **2** A 73-year-old man has anaemia, weight loss and difficulty swallowing.

☐ **3** A young man is complaining of violent retching after an alcoholic binge.

49 THEME: MEDIASTINAL MASSES

A   Anterior mediastinum
B   Middle mediastinum
C   Posterior mediastinum
D   Superior mediastinum

For each of the pathologies listed below, select the correct part of the mediastinum in which they are found from the above list. Each option may be used once, more than once, or not at all.

☐ **1** Thymic lesions

☐ **2** Neural tumours

☐ **3** Thyroid mass

☐ **4** Lymphoma

☐ **5** Bronchogenic cyst

50 THEME: HEART MURMURS

A   Continuous systolic murmur
B   Early diastolic murmur
C   Ejection systolic murmur
D   Machinery murmur
E   Split second heart sound

For each of the abnormalities below, choose the most likely diagnosis from the list of options above. Each option may be used once, more than once, or not at all.

☐ **1** Ventricular septal defect (VSD)

☐ **2** Atrial septal defect (ASD)

☐ **3** Aortic regurgitation

51 THEME: CHEST INJURY

A   Aortic injury
B   Flail segment
C   Pericardial injury
D   Pneumothorax
E   Pulmonary contusions

For each of the scenarios below, select the most likely chest injury from the list of options above. Each option may be used once, more than once, or not at all.

☐ **1** A young man with a penetrating chest injury is clinically well on admission, and has a normal chest film. However, he deteriorates while on the ward and has a tachycardia, hypotension and dyspnoea when reviewed. His pulse is weak and JVP is raised.

☐ **2** A cricketer is hit by a ball in the chest. He initially carries on with the game but then collapses, and is 'blue-lighted' to the Emergency Department. He is dyspnoeic, drowsy and has barely audible breath sounds.

52 THEME: CARDIAC PHYSIOLOGY

	HR	SV	Pulse pressure (PP)
A	40	250	40
B	50	140	50
C	100	70	70
D	120	35	70
E	180	25	90
F	200	35	50

Select the most appropriate set of observations from the above table for each of the cases below. Each option may be used once, more than once, or not at all.

☐ **1** A 25-year-old marathon runner is seen at preadmission clinic for elective surgery.

☐ **2** A 40-year-old patient presents with uncontrolled hyperthyroidism.

☐ **3** A fit 50-year-old patient undergoing laparoscopic cholecystectomy.

53 THEME: DYSPNOEA

A	Cardiac tamponade
B	Left haemothorax
C	Left tension pneumothorax
D	Pulmonary embolus

For each of the descriptions listed below, select the most likely diagnosis from the above list. Each option may be used once, more than once, or not at all.

☐ **1** A patient has distended neck veins, having been stabbed lateral to the trachea. Examination reveals decreased breath sounds, hyper-resonant lung fields and tracheal deviation.

☐ **2** A patient presents with ECG changes in lead III, Q wave with inverted T and changes in lead I.

☐ **3** A patient has dullness to percussion of the left chest.

54   THEME: MULTIPLE ENDOCRINE NEOPLASIA (MEN) SYNDROMES

A   MEN I
B   MEN IIA
C   MEN IIB

For each option given below, select the most likely MEN syndrome from the above list. Each option may be used once, more than once, or not at all.

☐ **1**   Submucosal neuromas

☐ **2**   Pancreatic islet-cell adenomas

☐ **3**   Marfanoid appearance

☐ **4**   Pituitary hyperplasia

Questions

55 THEME: UPPER ABDOMINAL PAIN

A	Biliary colic	G	Pancreatitis
B	Bleeding duodenal ulcer	H	Peptic ulcer
C	Bleeding gastric ulcer	I	Perforated duodenal ulcer
D	Cholecystitis	J	Perforated gastric ulcer
E	Gastritis	K	Perforated oesophagus
F	Leaking abdominal aortic aneurysm		

For each of the following situations, select the most likely cause of abdominal pain from the above list. Each option may be used once, more than once or not at all.

☐ **1** A 35-year-old man on steroids was admitted to accident and emergency (the Emergency Department) with hypotension and tachycardia. He was also noted to have a raised respiratory rate and low urine output. A history of back pain and some bruising was noted in the flanks.

☐ **2** A 43-year-old lady presented to the Emergency Department with an 8-week history of epigastric discomfort, she had a pyrexia 38 °C and a WBC 15×10^9/l. There was associated nausea but no vomiting or features of generalised peritonitis. There was some indication of increased pain on ingestion of fatty foods.

☐ **3** A 65-year-old man was admitted to the Emergency Department with sudden onset of upper abdominal pain and vomiting. He had drunk 4 pints of beer the night before. On examination there is resonance on percussion over the liver.

36

56 THEME: RIGHT ILIAC FOSSA PAIN

A	Appendicitis	E	Perforated duodenal ulcer
B	Ectopic pregnancy	F	Ruptured ovarian cyst
C	Irritable bowel syndrome	G	Terminal ileal Crohn's disease
D	Ovarian torsion	H	Ureteric stone

For each of the following situations below, select the most likely cause of the pain from the above list. Each item may be used once, more than once, or not at all.

☐ **1** A 28-year-old woman developed sudden onset of pain in the right iliac fossa. Pain was improved by walking around the examination room in the Emergency department.

☐ **2** A 28-year-old woman presents with recurrent abdominal pain localised mostly to the right iliac fossa. She opens her bowels four times a day. The stool was noted to be of liquid consistency. Pain was reported to be worse when eating but relieved by bowel movement. A loss of 5 kg in weight was noted.

57 THEME: TREATMENTS FOR ANAL PAIN

A	Anal canal carcinoma	F	Proctitis secondary to
B	Fissure in ano		Crohn's disease
C	Low subcutaneous anal fistula	G	Radiation proctitis
	(below the dentate line)	H	Solitary rectal ulcer syndrome
D	Perianal abscess	I	Transphincteric anal fistula
E	Perianal haematoma		with supralevator extension

For each of the treatment options, select the most likely answer from the above list. Each option may be used once, more than once, or not at all.

☐ **1** Biofeedback

☐ **2** 4% Formalin (topical)

☐ **3** Insertion of seton

☐ **4** 2% Diltiazem ointment

☐ **5** Botulinum toxin

58 THEME: ABDOMINAL SYSTEM INVESTIGATIONS

A	Barium enema	F	Flexible sigmoidoscopy
B	Colonoscopy	G	MRI
C	CT	H	Red cell scan
D	Endoanal ultrasound	I	Single contrast gastrografin
E	Evacuation proctogram		enema

For each of the following scenarios, select the most likely answer from the above list. Each option may be used once, more than once, or not at all.

☐ **1** Family history of colonic cancer: brother (aged 35 years), sister (aged 32 years) and father (aged 60 years).

☐ **2** An 88-year-old lady with a change in bowel habit.

☐ **3** A 25-year-old man with bright red rectal bleeding.

☐ **4** Angiodysplasia of the colon.

59 THEME: ABDOMINAL SYSTEM INVESTIGATIONS

A	Colonoscopy	F	Mesenteric angiogram
B	CT	G	MRI
C	Endoanal ultrasound	H	Red cell scan
D	Evacuation proctogram	I	Single contrast gastrografin
E	Flexible sigmoidoscopy		enema

For each of the following scenarios, select the most likely answer from the above list. Each option may be used once, more than once, or not at all.

☐ **1** Local invasiveness of rectal cancer in the pelvis.

☐ **2** Evidence of secondary spread to the liver.

☐ **3** A 35-year-old lady with passive and urge faecal incontinence following obstetric injury.

60 THEME: TIMING OF SURGICAL PROCEDURES

A   Urgent operation within next 12–24 hours
B   Wait 2 weeks and operate
C   Wait 6 months and operate
D   Wait 6 weeks and operate

For each of the following scenarios, select the most likely answer from the above list. Each option may be used once, more than once, or not at all.

☐ **1**   A 45-year-old lady is brought to the Emergency Department with an 18-hour history of right upper quadrant pain, and a tender mass in this region. Temperature is 39 °C and ultrasound demonstrates a distended gallbladder with pericholecystic fluid. The WBC count is 26 × 10^9/l. The patient remains pyrexial and tachycardic after 24 hours of antibiotics.

☐ **2**   A 12-year-old boy is brought to the Emergency Department with a 3-day history of right iliac fossa pain. There is a palpable mass with only localised tenderness. Temperature and pain respond to intravenous antibiotics.

☐ **3**   A 34-year-old lady with known Crohn's disease of the terminal ileum undergoes a right hemicolectomy. Unfortunately, 9 days post-operation she develops two enterocutaneous fistulas. She is otherwise well.

☐ **4**   A 79-year-old man is admitted with a sigmoid perforation secondary to diverticular disease. He had a Hartmann's procedure and makes a satisfactory post-operative recovery. He is extremely keen for a reversal and asks when this procedure might be feasible.

61 THEME: RECTAL BLEEDING

A	Anal carcinoma	G	Diverticular disease
B	Anal fissure	H	Haemorrhoids
C	Angiodysplasia	I	Infective colitis
D	Colonic carcinoma	J	Ischaemic colitis
E	Colonic polyp	K	Ulcerative colitis
F	Crohn's disease		

For each of the following scenarios, select the most likely answer from the above list. Each option may be used once, more than once, or not at all.

☐ **1** A 20-year-old lady presents with a 3-week history of bright red rectal bleeding associated with pain on defaecation. Her symptoms started post-partum.

☐ **2** A 32-year-old man presents with a 1-week history of colicky lower abdominal pain. This is associated with bloody diarrhoea, increased stool frequency and weight loss. A mass is palpable in the right iliac fossa. He is anaemic and has a CRP of 200.

☐ **3** A 37-year-old homosexual presents with a 3-month history of episodes of bright red rectal bleeding associated with pain and itching. On examination he has an area of ulceration at the anal verge with an everted irregular edge.

62 THEME: POST-OPERATIVE PYREXIA

A Anastomotic leak	F Respiratory tract infection
B Basal atelectasis	G Subphrenic abscess
C Deep-vein thrombosis	H Urinary tract infection
D Pelvic abscess	I Wound infection

For each of the following situations, select the most likely answer from the above list. Each option may be used once, more than once, or not at all.

☐ **1** A 10-year-old boy had an appendicectomy for perforated gangrenous appendicitis 3 days ago, with an uneventful post-operative recovery. He now returns to the Emergency Department with further lower abdominal pain and a swinging pyrexia of 39 °C. The wound is clean but there is tenderness on digital rectal examination.

☐ **2** An 81-year-old woman undergoes a laparotomy and a small bowel resection because of intra-abdominal adhesions. She has a prolonged recovery and is still being catheterised at day 14 post-operatively because of poor mobilisation. She has a temperature of 38.7 °C. There is no cough or GI symptoms and she is eating and drinking normally.

☐ **3** A 68-year-old man undergoes an anterior resection for rectal cancer. Post-operatively (day 5), he develops lower abdominal pain. On examination he looks flushed with a temperature of 38 °C and has low urine output.

☐ **4** A 70-year-old man undergoes a laparotomy with oversew of a perforated duodenal ulcer. Post-operatively (day 5) he develops a pyrexia of 38.6 °C with rigors. Clinical examination reveals some tenderness in the right upper quadrant. Crackles are heard at the right base and there is a small right pleural effusion on chest X-ray.

63 THEME : SCROTAL PAIN AND SWELLINGS

A	Epididymo-orchitis	F	Testicular teratoma
B	Hydrocele	G	Testicular torsion
C	Inguinoscrotal hernia	H	Torsion hydatid of Morgagni
D	Mumps	I	Varicocele
E	Testicular seminoma		

For each of the following situations, select the most likely cause of scrotal pain from the above list. Each option may be used once, more than once, or not at all.

☐ **1** A 20-year-old man has a 24-hour history of severe left scrotal pain and swelling. There is frequency of micturition and dysuria for the past few days. He has a temperature of 39 °C. There are leukocytes in the urine and the WBC is $15 \times 10^9/l$.

☐ **2** A 30-year-old man gives a history of dull left-sided scrotal pain for several months. On examination both testes are normal and you notice some veins on his scrotal skin. There is, however, a left hemiscrotal swelling present on lying down and it is not possible to get above this.

☐ **3** A 30-year-old man presents to his GP with swelling of his right–left hemiscrotum. He has noticed a dull ache but feels otherwise well. The testis is slightly enlarged and feels irregular in shape. Blood tests show raised β-HCG but normal α-fetoprotein.

☐ **4** A 7-year-old boy presents with a swelling of his right–left hemiscrotum. He is in considerable discomfort with a temperature of 37.5 °C. On examination his pain is very well localised to the upper pole of the testicle. A bluish hue can be seen through the scrotal skin.

64 THEME: SUTURE MATERIAL

A	'0'Vicryl	E	2'0' Prolene
B	3'0' PDS	F	2'0' Silk
C	6'0' PDS	G	1 PDS
D	6'0' Prolene	H	Stainless steel wire

For each of the following situations, select the most appropriate suture material for the procedure from the above list. Each option may be used once, more than once, or not at all.

☐ **1** Small bowel anastomosis.

☐ **2** Mid-line abdominal wound closure.

☐ **3** Sternotomy wound.

☐ **4** Distal end of a below-knee femoropopliteal bypass.

☐ **5** Securing a prosthetic mesh for incisional hernia repair.

Questions

65 THEME: DYSPHAGIA

A	Achalasia	F	Pharyngeal pouch
B	Diffuse oesophageal spasm	G	Plummer–Vinson syndrome
C	Oesophageal carcinoma	H	Retrosternal goitre
D	Para-oesophageal hernia	I	Syringomyelia
E	Pharyngeal palsy	J	Systemic sclerosis

For each of the following situations, select the most appropriate cause for dysphagia from the above list. Each option may be used once, more than once, or not at all.

☐ **1** A 32-year-old lady presents with intermittent dysphagia for solids and liquids, which is exacerbated by stress. She also gives a history of delayed regurgitation of food. There is no gastric air bubble seen on plain radiography and chest X-ray reveals a double right heart border.

☐ **2** A 57-year-old man (an ex-smoker) presents with an 8-month history of progressive dysphagia, retrosternal discomfort and cough during eating. He also had pneumonia recently and on examination, a lymph node is palpable in the cervical region.

☐ **3** An 81-year-old man presents with dysphagia, weight loss and occasional hoarseness of voice. On examination, there is a swelling in the anterior triangle of the neck.

☐ **4** A 65-year-old man presents with intermittent dysphagia for solids and liquids, and episodes of retrosternal chest pain. The pain radiates to the jaws and the interscapular region. Barium swallow reveals an area of intense muscle contraction mid-oesophagus.

Questions

66 THEME: ABDOMINAL PATHOLOGIES

A   Carcinoma of the ileo-caecal region
B   Carcinoma of the rectum
C   Crohn's disease
D   Diverticular disease
E   Endometriosis
F   Mesenteric infarction
G   Mittelschmerz
H   Ruptured ectopic pregnancy
I   Torsion of the ovary
J   Ulcerative colitis

For each of the following situations, select the most appropriate cause of the acute abdomen from the above list. Each option may be used once, more than once, or not at all.

☐ **1** A 73-year-old woman presents to the Emergency Department with lower abdominal distension and pain relieved by passing flatus. She also gives a history of altered bowel habit, a sense of incomplete evacuation, and blood mixed with her stools.

☐ **2** A 30-year-old smoker presents to the surgical outpatient clinic with a 4-month history of diarrhoea and abdominal colic. The patient has lost weight and has recently noted some mouth ulcers. A blood test reveals microcytic, hypochromic anaemia.

☐ **3** A 21-year-old lady is brought to the Emergency Department with severe generalised lower abdominal pain. She is pale, tachycardic, and her blood pressure is 90/54 mmHg.

☐ **4** An 83-year-old woman presents with a 12-hour history of severe generalised abdominal pain associated with nausea and vomiting. Her blood pressure is 100/70 mmHg. She is in atrial fibrillation and her bowel sounds are absent.

67 THEME: ACUTE ABDOMINAL PAIN

A Acute appendicitis	G Perforated peptic ulcer
B Acute cholecystitis	H Ruptured abdominal aortic
C Acute pancreatitis	aneurysm
D Biliary colic	I Ruptured liver
E Intestinal obstruction	J Ruptured spleen
F Obstructive jaundice	

For each of the following situations, select the most appropriate cause of acute abdominal pain from the above list. Each option may be used once, more than once, or not at all.

☐ **1** A 43-year-old barmaid complains of severe epigastric/right upper quadrant (RUQ) pain 2 hours after eating a meal of chips and fried chicken. The pain radiates to her back and makes her nauseated. There are no other systemic symptoms.

☐ **2** A 38-year-old executive of Asian origin is brought to the Emergency Department after his car was involved in a high-speed RTA. He presents with upper abdominal distension, guarding and signs of shock. He also complains of left shoulder tip pain and his past medical history includes recurrent episodes of malaria.

☐ **3** A 78-year-old lady presents with severe abdominal pain and signs of peritonism. She is on non-steroidal anti-inflammatory agents (NSAIDs) for rheumatoid arthritis. On examination, bowel sounds are absent. Erect chest X-ray shows free gas under the diaphragm.

☐ **4** A 74-year-old man is brought to the Emergency Department with sudden onset of upper abdominal and periumbilical pain radiating to his back. He is sweating, nauseated and feeling faint. His BP is 90/60 mmHg and his pulse rate is 110/min.

68 THEME: CHEST AND THORACIC WALL INJURIES

A	Cardiac tamponade	F	Perforated oesophagus
B	Diaphragmatic rupture	G	Pulmonary contusion
C	Flail chest	H	Ruptured thoracic aorta
D	Fracture of the sternum	I	Tension pneumothorax
E	Myocardial contusion	J	Traumatic haemothorax

For each of the following situations, select the most appropriate cause for the chest condition from the above list. Each option may be used once, more than once, or not at all.

☐ **1** A 38-year-old man presents with respiratory distress, tachycardia and distended neck veins following a penetrating injury to the right side of his chest. The patient's BP is 100/60 mmHg and respiratory rate is 20/min.

☐ **2** A 47-year-old taxi driver involved in a RTA presents with lacerations over his chest and abdomen. On examination, bowel sounds are heard in the chest. X-ray reveals bowel gas shadows in his left lung fields.

☐ **3** A 78-year-old gentleman who is a known alcoholic presents with severe chest pain following an episode of vomiting blood. Chest X-ray reveals gas in the mediastinum and in the subcutaneous tissues.

☐ **4** A 38-year-old motorcyclist is brought to the Emergency Department following a major RTA. On examination, he has a raised JVP and muffled heart sounds. The patient's blood pressure is 100/84 mmHg and his pulses fade on inspiration.

69 THEME: SURGICAL INVESTIGATIONS

A	Abdominal CT scan	E	ERCP
B	Abdominal ultrasound	F	Gastrografin enema
C	Barium enema (double contrast)	G	Small bowel follow-through
D	Colonoscopy		

For each of the following scenarios, select the most appropriate investigation from the above list. Each option may be used once, more than once, or not at all.

☐ **1** Hepatic hydatid cyst

☐ **2** Uncomplicated diverticular disease of the colon

☐ **3** Sclerosing cholangitis

☐ **4** Choledocholithiasis

70 THEME: ABDOMINAL PAIN INVESTIGATIONS (DIAGNOSTIC)

A	Abdominal ultrasound	F	Erect chest X-ray
B	Angiography (mesenteric)	G	FBC
C	Barium enema	H	Serum amylase
D	Barium meal and follow-through	I	Supine abdominal X-ray
E	CT		

For each of the patients described below, select the most likely investigation from the list of options above. Each option may be used once, more than once, or not at all.

☐ **1** A 75-year-old female orthopaedic patient on steroids for COPD and diclofenac for pain presents with acute, sudden-onset epigastric pain.

☐ **2** A 70-year-old psychiatric patient presents with periumbilical discomfort, gross abdominal distension and absolute constipation but no vomiting.

☐ **3** A 34-year-old woman with severe asthma was started on steroids. She later presents with acute-onset epigastric pain and vomiting. On examination she has decreased bowel sounds, guarding and rigidity.

71 THEME: HERNIAS

A	Diaphragmatic hernia	E	Obturator hernia
B	Epigastric hernia	F	Perineal hernia
C	Gluteal hernia	G	Sciatic hernia
D	Lumbar hernia	H	Spigelian hernia

For each site of herniation below, select the most likely hernial type from the above list. Each answer may be used once, more than once, or not at all.

☐ **1** Linea alba

☐ **2** Obturator canal

☐ **3** Lesser sciatic notch

72 THEME: NON-MALIGNANT CUTANEOUS LUMPS

A	Dercum's disease	F	Necrobiosis lipoidica
B	Dermatofibroma	G	Sebaceous cyst
C	Dermoid cyst	H	Seborrhoeic keratosis
D	Linear epidermal naevus	I	Stucco keratosis
E	Lupus vulgaris	J	Xanthelasma

For each of the following situations, select the most appropriate cause for the lesions from the above list. Each option may be used once, more than once, or not at all.

☐ **1** A 19-year-old Asian girl presents with an 8-month history of facial oedema associated with multiple cutaneous, jelly-like nodular lesions over her face. The skin surrounding the lesion appears congested.

☐ **2** An 18-year-old girl presents to her GP with an inflamed, tender cyst over the nape of her neck. The cyst has a punctum. She has had similar lesions over this region in the past.

☐ **3** A 65-year-old farmer presents with multiple, raised, brown, greasy lesions over his face. The surface over the lesions shows a network of crypts.

☐ **4** A 25-year-old lady presents with an itchy, pigmented, freely mobile nodule over her right leg. The patient noticed this lesion after an insect bite 5 days ago.

73 THEME: CUTANEOUS MALIGNANCIES

A Actinic keratosis	F Giant congenital naevus
B Amelanotic melanoma	G Keratoacanthoma
C Basal cell carcinoma	H Lentigo maligna
D Bowen's disease	I Nodular melanoma
E Cutaneous malignant lymphoma	J Squamous cell carcinoma

For each of the following situations, select the most appropriate cause for the skin lesion from the above list. Each option may be used once, more than once, or not at all.

☐ **1** A 75-year-old woman presents with a brown pigmented patch over her right cheek, which has been present for 10 years. It has an irregular outline and is thickened with a discrete tumour nodule.

☐ **2** A 23-year-old woman presents with a raised and sharply delineated black patch over her right lower leg. It has a smooth surface but is itchy and bleeds occasionally.

☐ **3** A 73-year-old retired builder presents with a small, well-defined ulcer over his right eye which has a pearly rolled-out edge. He states that it appeared 6 months ago as a nodule with a shiny white surface.

☐ **4** A 68-year-old farmer presents with a 4-week history of a solitary, fleshy and elevated nodule over his right cheek. He says that it is growing rapidly and on examination, it has a central hyperkeratotic core.

74 THEME: UPPER LIMB NERVE INJURIES

A   Anterior interosseous nerve
B   Injury to the lower cord of brachial plexus
C   Injury to the upper cord of brachial plexus
D   Long thoracic nerve
E   Median nerve
F   Musculocutaneous nerve
G   Posterior interosseous nerve
H   Radial nerve
I   Suprascapular nerve
J   Ulnar nerve

For each of the following statements, select the most likely cause of nerve injury from the above list. Each option may be used once, more than once, or not at all.

☐ **1**   A 25-year-old motorcyclist is brought to the Emergency Department after an RTA. He complains of pain in the root of his neck; on examination, his right arm is adducted, internally rotated and extended at the elbow. There is loss of sensation along the outer aspect of the arm and forearm.

☐ **2**   A 40-year-old patient presents to the Emergency Department with carpal dislocation (confirmed radiologically). On examination, there is loss of sensation over the thumb, index and middle fingers.

☐ **3**   A 65-year-old is brought to the Emergency Department with a wrist drop and sensory loss over a small patch at the base of the thumb. X-rays shows a mid-humerus fracture.

☐ **4**   A 30-year-old presents to the Emergency Department with a deep laceration to his right wrist after he was involved in a fight in a pub. On examination, he is unable to pinch and has got loss of sensation over his little and ring fingers.

75 THEME: AORTIC BYPASS GRAFTING

A   Aortobifemoral bypass
B   Axillobifemoral bypass
C   Femoral-to-femoral crossover
D   Left iliac angioplasty
E   Left iliac angioplasty and femoral crossover

For each of the patients described below, select the procedure of choice from the list of options above. Each option may be used once, more than once, or not at all.

☐ **1** A 50-year-old man has a 50-yard (~45 m) claudication distance, with complete occlusion of the lower aorta, with patent femoral vessels.

☐ **2** A 79-year-old man with emphysema requires home oxygen. He has complete occlusion of the aorta, with patent femoral vessels. His toes appear gangrenous and dusky.

☐ **3** A 43-year-old postman, otherwise fit and well, who is a non-smoker presents with acute onset claudication in both feet – he is determined to go back to work. He has an aortic bifurcation block with good femoral run-off on both sides.

Questions

76 THEME: LOWER LIMB ISCHAEMIA

A   Below-knee amputation
B   Fasciotomy
C   Femorodistal bypass
D   Femoropopliteal bypass
F   Lifestyle changes only
G   Percutaneous balloon angioplasty
H   Tissue plasminogen activator (TPA) infusion (intra-arterial)

For each of the presentations below, select the most likely single treatment from the options listed above. Each option may be used once, more than once, or not at all.

☐ 1   A 65-year-old man presents with intermittent claudication of the left calf. His claudication distance is 50 yards (~45 m). Angiography demonstrates a 1.5-cm stenosis of the left superficial femoral artery.

☐ 2   A 73-year-old diabetic presents with critical ischaemia of the right lower leg. Angiography reveals extensive disease of the superficial femoral, popliteal and tibial arteries. Pulse-generated, run-off assessment indicates a good run-off in the posterior tibial artery.

☐ 3   A 72-year-old man presents with a 4-hour history of acute ischaemia of the left leg. Clinical examination demonstrates signs of acute ischaemia with no evidence of gangrene, mottling or neurological deficit. An urgent angiogram reveals a complete thrombotic occlusion of the distal superficial femoral artery.

☐ 4   A 57-year-old smoker has a history of intermittent claudication of his right calf. His claudication distance is 0.5 mile (~0.8 km). Angiography reveals a 12-cm stenosis in the proximal superficial femoral artery. This has had no effect on his lifestyle, work or social activities.

☐ 5   A 21-year-old motorcyclist presents with multiple injuries following a road traffic accident. Clinical examination reveals a critically ischaemic right lower leg. The right dorsalis pedis pulse is weak. His right calf is tense and swollen. The intracompartmental pressure is 55 mmHg. Angiography shows no discontinuity of the arterial tree.

77 THEME: LOWER LIMB VENOUS DISEASE

A   Compression bandaging
B   Elevation, rest, NSAIDs and antibiotics
C   Emergency surgery
D   IV heparin
E   Warfarinisation

For each of the patients described below, select the treatment of choice from the list of options above. Each option may be used once, more than once, or not at all.

☐ **1** A woman has thrombosed varicose veins and cellulitis.

☐ **2** A woman develops a swollen and tender left leg 5 days after surgery.

☐ **3** A 64-year-old woman, who is a known case of venous insufficiency, presents with hypotension and profuse bleeding from the medial malleolus of the right leg. Conservative treatment has failed.

78 THEME: CAROTID ARTERY DISEASE

A   Carotid angiogram
B   Carotid Doppler
C   CT scan
D   ECG

What initial investigation would you perform for each of the patients listed below? Each option may be used once, more than once, or not at all.

☐ **1** A 71-year-old man presents with a normal pulse, left carotid bruit and left TIAs.

☐ **2** A 71-year-old man presents with a normal pulse, left carotid bruit and a dense left hemiplegia.

79 THEME: INVESTIGATION OF CAROTID ARTERY DISEASE

A Carotid angiography
B CT scan of head
C Duplex Doppler ultrasound of carotid arteries
D Magnetic resonance angiography (MRA)
E Near-infrared spectroscopy
F Transcranial Doppler ultrasound

From each of the statements below, select the most appropriate investigation from the above list. Each option may be used once, more than once, or not at all.

☐ **1** What should be the initial investigation in a 65-year-old man presenting with an episode of amaurosis fugax affecting his right eye?

☐ **2** Which is the most appropriate investigation for a 28-year-old woman who collapses with a possible dense, right-sided stroke?

☐ **3** Which is the most appropriate procedure for intraoperative monitoring during carotid endarterectomy?

80 THEME: VASCULAR TUMOURS

A Angiosarcoma
B Chemodectoma
C Leiomyomas
D Glomus jugulare tumour
E Kaposi's sarcoma

Match the most appropriate feature above with the list below. Each option may be used once, more than once, or not at all.

☐ **1** Carotid artery

☐ **2** Rapid growing, bulky

☐ **3** Blue-red macule with HIV

☐ **4** Buzzing sensation in head

81 THEME: LEG ULCERS

A   Arterial
B   Diabetic
C   Neoplastic
D   Postphlebitic
E   Venous

For each of the patient scenarios below, select the aetiology of the most likely ulcer from the above list. Each option may be used once, more than once, or not at all.

☐ **1** A 72-year-old woman presents with a 2-year history of an intermittently healing, shallow ulcer above the right medial malleolus. The surrounding skin has a brown discoloration. Ten years previously, she was involved in an RTA and sustained pelvic fractures, which were treated with traction and bedrest.

☐ **2** A 68-year-old man presents with a deep, painless ulcer beneath the heel of his right foot, which has gradually deteriorated in the two months since his admission for pneumonia. The ulcer is surrounded by wet macerated skin and culture has grown MRSA and *Pseudomonas* species.

☐ **3** A 94-year-old man presents with a deep, painful ulcer at the tip of his great toe. He has gradually been getting less mobile over the last few months and the pain in his toe prevents him from sleeping.

82 THEME: CAROTID ARTERY DISEASE

A Carotid angiography
B Carotid duplex
C CT head
D MRI head
E Right carotid endarterectomy

For each of the patients described below, select the most likely intervention from the list of options above. Each option may be used once, more than once, or not at all.

☐ **1** A patient has a resolving right-sided CVA. A carotid duplex shows 99% stenosis of the left internal carotid artery and a completely occluded right internal carotid artery.

☐ **2** A 30-year-old patient with optic neuritis develops foot drop.

☐ **3** A resolving recent left-sided hemiparesis with 90% right internal carotid artery stenosis.

83 THEME: VARICOSE VEINS

A Compression and warfarin
B Elevation and NSAIDs
C IV heparin
D Varicose vein surgery

For each of the patients described below, select the most likely intervention from the list of above options. Each option may be used once, more than once, or not at all.

☐ **1** A 54-year-old man presents with varicose veins and a bleeding varicose ulcer.

☐ **2** A 30-year-old woman presents with varicose veins and an acute episode of thrombophlebitis.

☐ **3** A 45-year-old woman presents with varicose veins and a swollen leg. Duplex confirms a DVT.

84   THEME: LOWER LIMB ISCHAEMIA

A   Angioplasty
B   Aortofemoral bypass graft
C   Correct the risk factors and provide conservative treatment
D   Femoropopliteal bypass graft
E   Surgical embolectomy

Select the most appropriate option above for the treatment of the patients below. Each option may be used once, more than once, or not at all.

☐   **1**   A 55-year-old man presents with a sudden onset of severe pain in his left foot and calf. There is no preceding history of intermittent claudication but he experienced a myocardial infarction two weeks ago. He is unable to move his foot, which is now mottled and cold. There are absent pulses below his left knee but a palpable femoral pulse. ECG reveals Q waves with sinus rhythm.

☐   **2**   A 75-year-old man presents to the outpatient clinic with right buttock and thigh pain when walking 100 yards. He smokes 30 cigarettes per day and has a poor cardiac history (three previous MIs, hypertension and left ventricular failure). Ankle brachial Doppler pressure ratio in the right leg is 0.3 and that on the left 0.6. An arteriogram shows an isolated 3 cm 80% stenosis in the right common iliac artery with good run-off. There is evidence of 40% stenosis in the left superficial femoral artery with well-developed collaterals.

☐   **3**   A 65-year-old man presents with pain in his foot when at rest. He has given up smoking and is otherwise fit and well. Angiography shows a 10-cm block in the superficial femoral artery with good distal run-off.

85 THEME: 5-YEAR GRAFT PATENCY RATES

A   Aortobifemoral graft
B   Axillofemoral graft
C   Femoral–femoral crossover graft
D   Femoropopliteal PTFE graft patency (below knee)
E   Reversed vein femoropopliteal graft

For each of the percentages below, select the most likely single graft from the options listed above. Each option may be used once, more than once, or not at all.

☐ **1** 70%

☐ **2** 80%

☐ **3** 60%

☐ **4** 35%

☐ **5** 90%

86 THEME: LOWER LIMB ULCERATION

A	Basal cell carcinoma	F	Pyoderma gangrenosum
B	Erythema nodosum	G	Sickle cell disease
C	Hypertensive ulcer	H	Squamous cell carcinoma
	(Martorell's ulcer)	I	Vasculitic ulcer
D	Necrobiosis lipoidica	J	Venous ulcer
E	Neuropathic ulcer		

For each of the following profiles, select the most likely cause of the ulcer from the above list. Each option may be used once, more than once, or not at all.

☐ **1** A 54-year-old lady with known inflammatory bowel disease presents with a large nodulo-pustular ulcerating lesion over her right anterior shin. It has a blue overhanging necrotic edge. The arterial blood pressure index (ABPI) is normal.

☐ **2** A 57-year-old obese lady with varicose veins presents with a large ulcer over her left medial malleolus. This is associated with surrounding lipodermatosclerosis and eczema. The ABPI in this leg is 1.05.

☐ **3** A 59-year-old man presents with ulceration over the distal tips of three toes in his left foot and over his right heel. He also complains of paraesthesia in both his feet. The ABPI is 1.02 on the right and 1.16 on the left. On neurological assessment, proprioception and vibration sense are reduced.

☐ **4** A 30-year-old Afro-Caribbean lady presents with a 4-month history of a painful ulcer over her right shin. ABPIs are normal. She is anaemic and has mild splenomegaly.

87 THEME: RENAL TRANSPLANT

| A | Acute rejection | C | Chronic rejection |
| B | Blood group mismatch | D | Hyperacute rejection |

Match the following concerning transplantation. Each option may be used once, more than once, or not at all.

☐ **1** The humoral system is responsible for this.

☐ **2** Cellular immunity is responsible for this.

☐ **3** This causes haemolysis.

☐ **4** Pre-sensitisation is responsible for this.

88 THEME: PAEDIATRIC INVESTIGATIONS

A	A 'cone' on contrast enema
B	A 'double-bubble sign' on plain abdominal X-ray (AXR)
C	A 'target' lesion on abdominal ultrasound
D	A type-II curve on a diuretic renogram
E	Air-filled cysts in the left chest
F	Clubbed renal calyces on a micturating cystogram
G	Hypochloraemic metabolic alkalosis
H	Intramural gas on plain AXR

For each of the clinical scenarios below, select the most appropriate feature on investigation from the above list. Each option may be used once, more than once, or not at all.

☐ **1** A 10-hour-old term baby presents with persistent bile-stained vomiting.

☐ **2** A 10-day-old baby, born at 30 weeks, presents with bile-stained vomiting and bloody diarrhoea.

☐ **3** An 8-month-old infant presents with colicky abdominal pain and bleeding per rectum.

☐ **4** A 2-day-old baby presents with abdominal distension, bile-stained vomiting and failure to pass meconium.

89 THEME: PAEDIATRIC CONDITIONS

A   Intussusception
B   Meckel's diverticulum
C   Pyloric stenosis
D   Replicated bowel

For each of the patients described below, select the most likely diagnosis from the list of options above. Each option may be used once, more than once, or not at all.

☐ **1** A 2-year-old presents with bilious vomiting, bleeding per rectum and a sausage-shaped mass in the abdomen.

☐ **2** A 2-month-old presents with non-bilious projectile vomiting after feeds.

☐ **3** A 5-year-old presents with bilious vomiting and bleeding per rectum.

90 THEME: NEONATAL SURGICAL DIAGNOSES

A	Duodenal atresia	F	Mid-gut volvulus
B	Exomphalos	G	Necrotising enterocolitis (NEC)
C	Gastroschisis	H	Oesophageal atresia
D	Hirschsprung's disease	I	Tracheo-oesophageal fistula
E	Imperforate anus		

For each of the clinical scenarios given below, select the most likely diagnosis from the above list. Each option may be used once, more than once, or not at all.

☐ **1** A male infant with trisomy 21, born at term, presents with abdominal distension, bile-stained vomiting and collapse. There has been no passage of meconium.

☐ **2** An antenatal observation of intestine and liver outside the fetal abdomen.

☐ **3** A previously well male infant, 6 weeks old and born at 35 weeks gestation, presents with bile-stained vomiting.

☐ **4** A 4-hour-old female infant noted to be 'frothy', was born to a mother with polyhydramnios during pregnancy.

☐ **5** An 8-day-old female infant presents with respiratory distress at each oral feed.

91 THEME: PAEDIATRIC NEWBORN GASTROINTESTINAL
    DISORDERS

A	Biliary atresia	E	Meconium ileus
B	Duodenal atresia	F	Necrotising enterocolitis
C	Hirschsprung's disease	G	Pyloric stenosis
D	Intussusception		

**For each of the patients described below, select the most likely diagnosis
from the list of options above. Each option may be used once, more than
once, or not at all.**

☐ **1** A 3-day-old child presents with a scaphoid abdomen, and is unable
to feed with bilious vomiting.

☐ **2** A 10-day-old child presents with a right abdominal mass and
distension, with a history of passing meconium for only three days
with the help of suppositories. He is now passing blood per rectum.

☐ **3** A baby presents needing enemas to open its bowels owing to a
24-hour delay in passing meconium.

92 THEME: GASTROINTESTINAL DISORDERS IN NEONATES

A	Ano-rectal atresia	F	Meckel's diverticulum
B	Hirschsprung's disease	G	Meconium ileus
C	Infantile hypertrophic	H	Mid-gut malrotation
	pyloric stenosis	I	Necrotising enterocolitis
D	Intestinal atresia	J	Tracheo-oesophageal fistula
E	Intussusception	K	Volvulus neonatorum

For each of the following situations, select the most appropriate cause of diarrhoea/vomiting from the above list. Each option may be used once, more than once, or not at all.

☐ **1** An 8-month-old male baby with haemophilia presents with intermittent episodes of inconsolable crying and vomiting. The parents say the baby's stools are mixed with blood. On examination, a mass is palpable over the right side of abdomen.

☐ **2** A new-born baby girl with cystic fibrosis presents with gross abdominal distension and bilious vomiting. Abdominal X-ray shows distended coils of bowel, but no fluid levels. Rectal examination reveals an empty rectum.

☐ **3** A premature infant (30-week gestation) presents with bloody diarrhoea, and a distended and tense abdomen. On examination, there is erythema over the anterior abdominal wall. The infant also manifests signs of sepsis.

☐ **4** A newborn baby boy presents with mild abdominal distension, bilious vomiting, and failure to pass meconium after 24 hours. Plain abdominal X-ray reveals dilated loops of bowel with fluid levels and barium enema demonstrates a 'conical appearance' in a segment of the colon.

93 THEME: DISORDERS OF BONE

A	Achondroplasia	F	Osteogenesis imperfecta
B	Craniocleidodysostosis	G	Osteopetrosis
C	Diaphyseal aclasis	H	Perthe's disease
D	Ollier's disease	I	Rickets
E	Osteochondrodystrophy	J	Scurvy

For each of the following situations, select the most appropriate cause for the presentation from the above list. Each option may be used once, more than once, or not at all.

☐ **1** A 13-year-old boy is brought to the orthopaedic outpatient clinic with a history of tiredness, recurrent throat and chest infections and gradual loss of hearing. X-ray reveals a 'marble bone' appearance.

☐ **2** A 14-year-old boy, who is small for age, is brought to his GP with loss of hearing in both ears. On examination, he has a blue sclera, knock-knees, and hypermobile fingers. X-rays show multiple fractures (old) of the long bones and irregular patches of ossification.

☐ **3** A 3-year old boy is brought to the GP surgery with a swollen and painful right knee joint. The parents also say that they recently noticed some bleeding from his gums. He lies still and refuses to move the limb. X-ray shows generalised rarification of the bones in his legs.

☐ **4** A 2-year-old infant is brought to the Emergency Department with convulsions. On examination, the child lies listless and flaccid, appears small for age and there is noticeable thickening of both wrists. X-ray shows an increase in the depth and width of the epiphysis of the lower ends of the radius and ulna.

94 THEME: PELVIC FRACTURE

A   Rotationally and vertically stable
B   Rotationally unstable, vertically stable pelvic fracture
C   Rotationally unstable, vertically unstable pelvic fracture

For each of the pelvic injuries below, select the correct classification of pelvic fracture from the above list. Each option may be used once, more than once, or not at all.

☐ **1** Lateral compression fracture

☐ **2** Open-book fracture

☐ **3** Vertical shear injuries

☐ **4** Isolated iliac wing fracture

☐ **5** Isolated pubic ramus fracture

95 THEME: PERIPHERAL NERVE ANATOMY

A	Axillary	F	Radial
B	Long thoracic	G	Suprascapular
C	Medial pectoral	H	Thoracodorsal
D	Median	I	Ulnar
E	Musculocutaneous	J	Upper subscapular

For each of the patients listed below, select the nerve most likely to be involved from the above list. Each option may be used once, more than once, or not at all.

☐ **1** While playing football, a young man dislocates his right shoulder. The dislocation is reduced soon after. Once the shoulder is pain-free, he notices that he cannot carry weights with his right arm and is unable to raise his arm from his side for more than a few degrees. Neurological examination reveals loss of abduction and blunted sensation over the skin covering the lateral part of the deltoid muscle. All reflexes are normal.

☐ **2** After a mastectomy, a 40-year-old woman loses the ability to fold her right arm behind her back and reach up to the opposite scapula.

☐ **3** A 15-year-old boy riding in the passenger seat of a car escapes any apparent injury after a head-on collision because he was wearing a seat belt. However, after the accident he was unable to raise his arm easily and has visited the Emergency Department twice with spontaneous dislocation of the shoulder.

☐ **4** A builder falls off a scaffolding on to his right side, fracturing his right humerus. Because of the patient's shocked state and the pain, only a limited neurological examination is possible. This reveals an absence of the brachioradialis reflex, blunted cutaneous sensation over the first dorsal interosseous muscle and wrist drop.

☐ **5** After a radical mastectomy, a 41-year-old woman is unable to push a loaded supermarket trolley with her right arm. Her husband has noticed a deformity in her upper back on the right side that becomes more prominent when she pushes against resistance with the outstretched right arm.

96 THEME: SHOULDER PAIN

A   Acromioclavicular joint disruptions
B   Biceps rupture
C   Subacromial bursitis
D   Supraspinatus rupture
E   Supraspinatus tendonitis

For each of the patients described below, choose the most suitable diagnosis from the list of options above. Each option may be used once, more than once, or not at all.

☐ **1** A 52-year-old plasterer complains of a 1-year history of shoulder pain and difficulty in lifting his arm up while performing his job. On examination, he had marked tenderness over the acromium. He has to bend over to the affected side to initiate shoulder abduction. He has no difficulty in passive abduction of his arm.

☐ **2** A 32-year-old man presents with a 1-month history of shoulder pain especially on lifting the arm. On examination he has marked tenderness lateral to the acromial process with a painful arc of 60–120°.

97 THEME: LOW BACK PAIN

A	Discitis	E	Osteoporotic collapse
B	Facet joint arthrosis	F	Prolapsed intervertebral disc
C	Metastatic disease	G	Spondylolisthesis
D	Muscle strain		

For each of the clinical situations described below, please select the most likely diagnosis from the above list. Each option may be used once, more than once, or not at all.

☐ **1** A teenage boy presents to his GP with a 6-month history of increasing pain and stiffness in his lower lumbar spine. There is no history of trauma although he is an active sportsman. His lumbar spine is stiff on examination and there is bilateral limitation of straight leg raising with pain in the hamstring muscles.

☐ **2** A young man wakes up one morning complaining of pain in his lower back. The day before he had been redecorating his bedroom. There are no nerve root signs but his back is very stiff.

☐ **3** An active 88-year-old woman has had some back pain since she stumbled over her own doorstep 6 weeks ago. Her back was initially stiff but she feels there has been some improvement over the last 2 weeks.

☐ **4** A 3-year-old baby girl refuses to walk. Her symptoms began last night and she is irritable and unwell. Examination of her lower limbs is entirely normal but percussion of her lumbar spine causes her to cry.

☐ **5** A 45-year-old man gives a 3-month history of low back pain, which has become progressively worse such that he is now in agony and cannot get comfortable. The pain radiates to both buttocks and neurological examination suggests there are problems with the sacral nerve roots.

98 THEME: COMPLICATIONS OF HIP SURGERY

A   Death
B   Deep-vein thrombosis, no prophylaxis
C   Pulmonary embolus, no prophylaxis
D   Urinary retention, male
E   Wound infection without prophylaxis

Match the post-operative risk with the complication for hip replacement. Each option may be used once, more than once, or not at all.

☐ **1**   5–10%

☐ **2**   < 1%

☐ **3**   1–5%

☐ **4**   60%

☐ **5**   10–20%

99 THEME: KNEE INJURIES

A	Anterior cruciate rupture	D	Medial ligament rupture
B	Haemarthrosis	E	Patellar fracture
C	Injury to the medial meniscus	F	Tibial plateau fracture

For each of the clinical situations described below, select the most likely diagnosis from the above list. Each option may be used once, more than once, or not at all.

☐ **1** A 29-year-old man was hit by a car as he ran across the road. He was subsequently unable to weight-bear. His knee was bruised, swollen and tender.

☐ **2** A 45-year-old woman stumbled over an uneven paving stone and landed heavily on her knee. She walked aided into the Emergency Department with a swollen painful knee and was unable to straight leg raise.

☐ **3** A footballer sustained a twisting injury to his flexed knee while playing a game yesterday. He was unable to complete the game and by this morning his knee was very swollen. He was unable to fully flex or extend his knee.

☐ **4** A 25-year-old man landed awkwardly having jumped for a ball in the line-out during a rugby match. He heard a pop and was unable to complete the game. He noticed his knee swell immediately.

☐ **5** A 25-year-old man was involved in a tackle during a football game today. A valgus force was applied to the knee – he fell to the ground and noted that his knee was at a 'funny angle'. He has been unable to weight-bear and says that his knee feels 'unsafe'. On examination, his knee is generally tender, there is significant laxity on valgus stress but no definite effusion.

100 THEME: HEAD INJURY

A	Basal skull fracture	F	Haematoma of the scalp
B	Brain concussion	G	Open skull fracture
C	Compound skull fracture	H	Subaponeurotic haematoma
D	Diffuse axonal injury	I	Subarachnoid haemorrhage
E	Extradural haematoma	J	Subdural haematoma

For each of the following profiles, select the most likely cause of the condition from the above list. Each option may be used once, more than once, or not at all.

☐ **1** A 25-year-old motorcyclist is brought to the Emergency Department after being involved in a high speed RTA. He is unconscious and is noted to have a periorbital haematoma and bruising over the mastoid process. On examination, thin fluid mixed with blood is seen coming out of his nostrils.

☐ **2** A 39-year-old man walks into the Emergency Department after being assaulted with a baseball bat. He had a momentary loss of consciousness but feels fine at present. Skull X-ray reveals a linear fracture over his right parietal area. While in casualty, he suddenly becomes confused and later unconscious with a Glasgow coma scale (GCS) score of eight. His right pupil is dilated.

☐ **3** A 56-year-old man presents to the trauma clinic with a fluctuant swelling under his scalp and bilateral swollen eyelids. He fell off a 5-feet high step ladder 5 days ago. On examination, the swelling extents from the frontal to the occipital region. He is well otherwise and his GCS is 15.

☐ **4** A 54-year-old alcoholic is brought to the Emergency Department with a left-sided hemiparesis. He thinks he knocked his head against the bathtub 10 days ago. Since then he has had headaches and has been noticed to have a fluctuating level of consciousness.

Questions

101 THEME: JOINT AND BACK PAIN

A	Ankylosing spondylitis	F	Paget's disease
B	Intervertebral disc herniation	G	Reiter's syndrome
C	Metastatic disease	H	Rheumatoid arthritis G
D	Multiple myeloma	I	Spinal stenosis
E	Osteoarthritis	J	Spondylolisthesis

For each of the following statements, select the most likely cause of joint/back pain from the above list. Each option may be used once, more than once, or not at all.

☐ **1** A 25-year-old presents with an unstable fracture of the fourth lumbar vertebra following a fall. He is on long-term NSAIDs for a painful and stiff back. On examination, he has kyphosis and serology for human leukocyte antigen B27 (HLA-B27) is positive.

→☐ **2** A 33-year-old previously fit patient presents with an acute low backache, which commenced when he was lifting a heavy object at work. He also complains of shooting pain radiating down the back of his right thigh.

☐ **3** A 25-year-old presents with a painful right knee, and vesicles and pustules over the soles of his feet. He also complains of soreness in his eyes and burning on micturition. He gives a history of unprotected sex 2 months ago.

☐ **4** A 12-year-old gymnast is brought by her parents to the orthopaedic clinic with lower backache of 1-year duration. On examination, she has L5 root pain and a hamstring spasm. Straight leg raise is reduced.

102 THEME: LOWER LIMB PATHOLOGIES

A   Ascending lymphangitis
B   Common peroneal nerve palsy
C   Compartment syndrome
D   Deep-vein thrombosis
E   Elephantiasis
F   Haemarthrosis of the knee joint
G   Milroy's syndrome
H   Ruptured Achilles tendon
I   Superficial thrombophlebitis
J   Torn calf muscle

For each of the following statements, select the most likely cause of limb pain from the above list. Each option may be used once, more than once, or not at all.

☐ **1**   A 37-year-old motorcyclist is brought to the Emergency Department following an RTA. He complains of numbness in his foot and unremitting pain in his right lower leg which is made worse by passive dorsiflexion of his ankle. X-ray reveals a closed fracture of the right tibia.

☐ **2**   A 73-year-old patient presents with mild pyrexia, and pain and swelling in her left calf. She underwent total hip replacement 8 days ago.

☐ **3**   A 13-year-old adolescent is brought to her GP with a swollen right leg; the swelling is extending up to the knee. It is painless and the parents say that the swelling was first noticed shortly after menarche. She is otherwise systemically well.

☐ **4**   A 42-year-old teacher is persuaded to take part in a staff–student tennis match. She has not done any exercise in the last 10 years. While running for a ball, she experiences sudden, severe pain in her right calf and is unable to play any longer. On examination, there is swelling and tenderness just above the heel, and she is unable to walk tiptoe.

103 THEME: LOWER LIMB NERVE INJURY

A   Common peroneal nerve
B   Femoral nerve
C   Lateral cutaneous nerve of thigh
D   Lateral plantar nerve
E   Medial plantar nerve
F   Pudendal nerve
G   Saphenous nerve
H   Sciatic nerve
I   Sural nerve
J   Tibial nerve

For each of the following statements, select the most likely cause of nerve injury from the above list. Each option may be used once, more than once, or not at all.

☐ **1**   A 28-year-old patient (37 weeks pregnant) presents to her GP with pain and paraesthesia over the upper outer aspect of her left thigh. She is able to walk and there is no restriction of movements in her hips or knees.

☐ **2**   A 32-year-old motorcyclist is brought to the Emergency Department after being involved in an RTA. He is unable to dorsiflex and evert his left foot. He has also reduced sensation over the lateral aspect of his lower leg and the dorsum of this foot. X-ray shows a fracture of the fibular neck.

☐ **3**   A 27-year-old man is brought to the Emergency Department following a gunshot injury to his right thigh. He has numbness over the anterior thigh and medial aspect of his leg. He is unable to extent his knee and the knee jerk is diminished.

☐ **4**   A 75-year-old patient presents to the orthopaedic outpatient clinic with a right foot drop and decreased sensation below the knee on the lateral side. He had a right total hip replacement 8 weeks ago.

Questions

104 THEME: BONE AND CONNECTIVE TISSUE TUMOURS

A	Chondrosarcoma	F	Osteochondroma
B	Ewing's sarcoma	G	Osteoclastoma
C	Fibrosarcoma	H	Osteoid osteoma
D	Leiomyosarcoma	I	Osteosarcoma
E	Malignant giant cell tumour	J	Rhabdomyosarcoma

For each of the following statements, select the most likely cause of pain/swelling from the above list. Each option may be used once, more than once, or not at all.

☐ **1** A 65-year-old presents with a swelling and pain over her left proximal humerus. The pain is worse at night. She also gives a history of weight loss. She has a raised ESR and she is undergoing treatment for Paget's disease.

☐ **2** A 13-year-old adolescent is brought by his parents to the GP with loss of weight, pain and fever. On examination, a soft but tender, ill-defined mass is palpable over his mid-thigh region.

☐ **3** A 23-year-old presents with mild discomfort and a lump over his right knee. He accidentally discovered the lump one week ago. On examination, it is bony hard and non-tender. He is systemically well.

☐ **4** A 28-year-old lady presents with weight loss, fever and a swelling over her right knee of a few weeks duration. Movements of her knee are severely restricted. X-ray reveals thinning of the cortex and a fracture of the distal femur. An extraosseous soft tissue mass is seen on MRI scan.

105 THEME: SHOULDER JOINT PATHOLOGIES

A   Acromioclavicular joint osteoarthritis
B   Acute supraspinatus tendonitis
C   Calcific tendonitis
D   Dislocated shoulder
E   Fracture of surgical neck of humerus
F   Frozen shoulder
G   Painful arc syndrome
H   Rotator cuff tear
I   Rupture of long head of biceps
J   Subdeltoid bursitis

For each of the following statements, select the most likely cause of shoulder pain from the above list. Each option may be used once, more than once, or not at all.

☐ **1** A 47-year-old lady presents with a 3-month history of painful shoulder. The pain is worse during the mid-phase of abduction and when bringing the hand down. There is no pain during the two extremes of movement.

☐ **2** A 60-year-old presents with a painful right shoulder after he fell off a tree 2 days ago. He has suffered from chronic shoulder pain in the past. On examination, there is tenderness at the tip of his shoulder and underneath the acromial process. He is unable to lift his arm and there is hunching of the shoulder.

☐ **3** A 68-year-old woman presents to her GP with an acutely painful left shoulder. There is no history of trauma. On examination, the shoulder joint is tender anterolaterally and there is restriction of all movements except external rotation. X-ray reveals radio-opaque deposits within the supraspinatus tendon.

☐ **4** A 23-year-old rugby player presents with sudden shoulder pain after being involved in a tackle during the game. On examination, there is loss of shoulder contour and a bulge is felt in the deltopectoral groove.

106 THEME: SPINAL PATHOLOGY

A   Acute disc prolapse
B   Scheuermann's disease
C   Spondylolisthesis
D   TB of the spine

For each of the patients listed below, select the diagnosis that best explains the clinical situation from the above list. Each option may be used once, more than once, or not at all.

☐ **1** An 18-year-old fast bowler and keen athlete presents with pain when extending his hip, he walks with scoliosis – acute onset.

☐ **2** A young immigrant from Bangladesh presents with lower back pain and fever.

107 THEME: NERVE DAMAGE

A   Horner's syndrome
B   Neurapraxia of the common peroneal nerve
C   Neurapraxia of the median nerve
D   Neurapraxia of the radial nerve
E   Neurotmesis of the common peroneal nerve
F   Neurotmesis of the medial nerve
G   Posterior interosseus nerve lesion
H   Sciatic nerve injury

For each of the patients listed below, select the site and type of nerve damage that best explains the clinical situation from the above list. Each option may be used once, more than once, or not at all.

□ **1** A 21-year-old man sustained a comminuted fracture of the right femur and a fracture of the ipsilateral tibia and fibula. He was treated with skeletal traction and a below-knee plaster overnight. On review it was noticed that he could not dorsiflex his right toes.

□ **2** A child falls on an outstretched hand and sustains a severely displaced supracondylar fracture of the humerus.

□ **3** Following a difficult elective plating of a non-union fracture of the humeral shaft, the patient was unable to extend his fingers and wrist. No nerves were visualised during the procedure.

□ **4** A motorcyclist came off his bike at considerable speed. Both he and his bike were then dragged down the road by a car. On examination he had a flail left upper limb.

□ **5** Following a total hip replacement performed via a posterior approach, the patient was noted to have a foot drop.

108 THEME: HAEMORRHAGIC SHOCK

A   Blood loss of 1.3 litres
B   Blood loss of 1.7 litres
C   Blood loss of 2.5 litres
D   Blood loss of 0.75 litre
E   Blood loss of 1 litre

For each of the above volumes of blood loss, select the most appropriate physiological change. Each option may be used once, more than once, or not at all.

☐ **1** Normal heart rate

☐ **2** Unconscious

☐ **3** Reduced systolic pressure

☐ **4** Confused and lethargic

☐ **5** Raised diastolic pressure

109 THEME: MICRO-ORGANISMS

A   *Clostridium difficile*
B   *Clostridium perfringens*
C   *Escherichia coli*
D   *Haemophilus influenzae*
E   *Staphylococcus aureus*
F   *Streptococcus pneumoniae*
G   None of the above

From the above list, choose the most common causative organism for the following infections. Each may be used once, more than once, or not at all.

☐ **1** Ludwig's angina

☐ **2** Vincent's angina

☐ **3** Post-operative diarrhoea

110 THEME: HEPATITIS B

A   HBsAg
B   Low titre of anti-HBs antibody
C   Positive HBeAg in serum
D   Raised titre of anti-HBs antibody

For each of the statements below, select the most likely answer from the above list. Each option may be used once, more than once, or not at all.

- [ ] **1** Requires a surgeon to immediately cease performing all invasive procedures.

- [ ] **2** Signifies previous hepatitis B infection.

- [ ] **3** Is produced after successful hepatitis B vaccination, indicating immunity.

- [ ] **4** Indicates current acute or chronic infection.

111 THEME: SKIN CONDITIONS

A   Erysipelas
B   Granuloma annulare
C   Necrotising fasciitis
D   Pyoderma gangrenosum
E   Pyogenic granuloma

For each of the patients described below, select the most likely diagnosis from the list of options above. Each option may be used once, more than once, or not at all.

- [ ] **1** A 55-year-old woman developed acute spreading cellulitis on one thigh, 1 week after drainage of a perianal abscess. She became ill with rigors and fever, and the affected skin appeared blistered.

- [ ] **2** A 5-year-old child presents with a red nodule on his lower lip, which bleeds easily on contact.

112 THEME: RENAL TRACT CALCULI

A Conservative management
B Extracorporeal shock wave lithotripsy (ESWL)
C Nephrectomy
D Percutaneous nephrolithotomy (PCNL)
E Percutaneous nephrostomy
F Ureteroscopy

For each of the patients below, select the most appropriate treatment from the above list. Each option may be used once, more than once, or not at all.

☐ **1** A 24-year-old woman presents with intermittent right loin pain. A mid-stream urine specimen (MSU) confirms microscopic haematuria. A plain radiograph shows a 1.2-cm calculus in the region of the right kidney. An intravenous urogram (IVU) confirms that it lies within the renal pelvis but is not causing obstruction.

☐ **2** A 45-year-old woman presents with a history of recurrent urinary tract infections (UTIs) and chronic left loin pain. An ultrasound shows a large echogenic mass in the left pelvicalyceal system. A plain kidney and upper bladder (KUB) demonstrates a staghorn calculus. A dimercaptosuccinic acid (DMSA) scan shows differential split function left : right, 9 : 91.

☐ **3** A 31-year-old man presents with colicky left loin pain. He is tachycardic, flushed and has a temperature of 38.5 °C. An IVU shows a 3-mm calculus in the mid-ureter.

113 THEME: BENIGN PROSTATIC HYPERPLASIA

A   Doxazosin
B   Prazosin
C   Radical prostatectomy
D   Retropubic (open) prostatectomy
E   Trial without catheter
F   Transurethral resection of the prostate (TURP)
G   Urethral catheterisation

For each of the patients below, select the most appropriate treatment from the above list. Each option may be used once, more than once, or not at all.

☐ **1** A 71-year-old man presents with acute urinary retention. On catheterisation his residual volume was 800 ml. His creatinine concentration on admission was 350 mmol/l. Following management of a postobstructive diuresis the creatinine concentration returned to 90 mmol/l. Digital rectal examination suggests a large benign prostate. A transrectal ultrasound shows a prostate volume of 180 ml with no hypoechoic areas.

☐ **2** A 56-year-old man presents with moderate lower urinary tract symptoms. He has persistent macroscopic haematuria. A digital rectal examination shows a large benign-feeling prostate. MSU, cytology, an IVU and flexible cystoscopy were negative for transitional cell carcinoma. He wishes to have another child in the near future.

☐ **3** A 59-year-old man presents with vague abdominal pain. An ultrasound showed bilateral hydronephrosis with a post-micturition residual volume of 1500 ml. His serum creatinine was normal.

114 THEME: TESTICULAR TUMOURS

A   Antiandrogen therapy
B   Chemotherapy
C   Close follow-up
D   Radical orchidectomy
E   Radiotherapy
F   Retroperitoneal lymph node dissection
G   Testicular biopsy

For each of the patients below, select the most appropriate subsequent treatment from the above list. Each option may be used once, more than once, or not at all.

☐ **1** A 34-year-old man presents with a hard, irregular swelling of his right testis. Alpha-fetoprotein and β-hCG are normal. An ultrasound shows a heterogeneous mass in the upper pole of the right testis. Investigations reveal no lymphadenopathy. A radical orchidectomy confirms a testicular seminoma which is completely excised.

☐ **2** A 22-year-old man presents with a hard, irregular swelling of his right testis. Ultrasound suggests a right testicular tumour and a left testis containing hypoechoic areas and microcalcification. A right radical orchidectomy and a left testicular biopsy are performed. Histology shows the right testicular seminoma is completely excised. A widespread, low-grade, intratubular, germ cell neoplasia is found on the left.

☐ **3** A 24-year-old man underwent an orchidectomy for a non-seminatous, germ cell tumour. A post-operative CT scan shows a 7-cm mass of retroperitoneal lymphadenopathy. After a course of chemotherapy the tumour markers normalise and CT scanning shows shrinkage of the nodal mass to 3.5 cm.

115 THEME: TRANSITIONAL CELL CARCINOMA

A Cystoscopy
B Intravesical BCG
C Intravesical mitomycin
D Methotrexate, doxorubicin, cyclophosphamide (M-VAC)
   chemotherapy
E Nephrectomy
F Nephroureterectomy
G Radical cystectomy
H Transurethral resection of bladder tumour

For each of the patients below, select the most appropriate treatment from the above list. Each option may be used once, more than once, or not at all.

☐ **1** A 64-year-old man presents with haematuria. An IVU shows normal upper tracts with a filling defect in the bladder. Flexible cystoscopy confirms a tumour.

☐ **2** A 58-year-old woman with a history of superficial bladder cancer is found to have an irregular filling defect in the right renal pelvis. CT confirms a solid mass.

☐ **3** A fit 55-year-old man presents with haematuria. Investigations reveal a bladder tumour. Transurethral resection of bladder tumour (TURBT) shows a muscle-invasive bladder cancer (stage T_2) and EUA confirms the bladder is mobile. CT scanning shows three 2–3-cm pelvic lymph nodes.

116 THEME: IMAGING

A	Cystogram	E	Plain KUB
B	DMSA scan	F	Retrograde ureterogram
C	DTPA scan	G	Spiral CT scan
D	IVU	H	Ultrasound

For each of the patients below, select the most appropriate treatment from the above list. Each option may be used once, more than once, or not at all.

☐ **1** A 34-year-old obese man presents with a sudden onset of colicky right loin pain radiating to his groin. He has microscopic haematuria. He has a history of severe anaphylaxis with intravenous contrast. An ultrasound scan is unhelpful because of obesity.

☐ **2** A 45-year-old woman has a right staghorn calculus on plain KUB. An IVU shows this kidney fails to excrete contrast. An ultrasound scan shows the kidney has a thin parenchyma without evidence of hydronephrosis.

☐ **3** A 22-year-old woman presents with a history of left loin pain shortly after drinking alcohol. An ultrasound scan shows hydronephrosis with a normal calibre ureter. An IVU shows a narrowing at the pelviureteric junction.

Questions

117 THEME: SCROTAL SWELLINGS

A	Acute epididymo-orchitis	F	Primary hydrocele
B	Chylocele	G	Strangulated inguinal hernia
C	Haematocele	H	Teratoma of testis
D	Lymph varix	I	Torsion of testis
E	Papillary cystoadenoma	J	Varicocele

For each of the following statements, select the most likely cause of scrotal pain from the above list. Each option may be used once, more than once, or not at all.

☐ **1** A 25-year-old presents with a painless, scrotal swelling of 8 months' duration which he attributes to an injury while playing football. On examination, the swelling over the testis is uniform, firm and smooth. There is loss of testicular sensation.

☐ **2** A 7-year-old presents with a sudden onset of severe pain in his right groin and lower abdomen associated with vomiting. On examination, a thickened and tender spermatic cord is palpable above the testis.

☐ **3** A 42-year-old tall, thin man of Asian origin presents with an aching pain and a left-sided scrotal swelling of 18 months duration. On examination, the scrotum on the left side hangs lower, cough impulse is present and the left testis is smaller than the right. The swelling disappears on lying down.

☐ **4** A 37-year-old presents with a right-sided scrotal swelling. On examination, the testis is not palpable and there is dullness on percussion. It is possible to get above the swelling.

118 THEME: RENAL PRESENTATIONS

A   Acute renal failure
B   Acute tubular necrosis
C   Focal segmental glomerulosclerosis
D   Gram-negative sepsis
E   Membranous glomerulonephritis
F   Renal abscess
G   Renal calculi
H   Renal papillary necrosis
I   Renal tubular acidosis
J   Renal tubular injury

For each of the following statements, select the most likely cause for the renal disease from the above list. Each option may be used once, more than once, or not at all.

☐ **1** A 32-year-old man presents to the Emergency Department with sudden excruciating right-sided abdominal pain of 4 hours duration. The pain is radiating from the right side of his ribs towards the groin. Urinalysis reveals red blood cells.

☐ **2** A 61-year-old presents with vomiting and anorexia of 4 days duration. He has had a left nephrectomy for chronic pyelonephritis 3 years ago and now suffers from recurrent right renal calculi. His urea is 24 and creatinine is 461.

☐ **3** A 46-year-old patient with AIDS is noted to have proteinuria, hypoalbuminaemia and generalised oedema 1 week after a renal transplant. Renal biopsy reveals IgM deposits in the glomerulus.

☐ **4** A 67-year-old man undergoes nephrostomy to relieve hydronephrosis of his right kidney. Four hours post-operatively, he develops rigors and pyrexia and his blood pressure is 100/60 mmHg.

119 THEME: RENAL TRACT PATHOLOGIES

A   Adenocarcinoma of the kidney
B   Adenoma of the renal cortex
C   Angioma of the renal artery
D   Angiomyolipoma
E   Nephroblastoma
F   Neuroblastoma
G   Papillary transitional cell tumour of the renal pelvis
H   Renal tuberculosis
I   Squamous cell carcinoma of the renal pelvis
J   Transitional cell carcinoma of the bladder
K   Transitional cell tumour of the ureter

For each of the following statements, select the most likely cause for renal tract disease from the above list. Each option may be used once, more than once, or not at all.

☐ **1**   A 55-year-old smoker presents with a dragging discomfort in his left loin. He also gives a history of haematuria with occasional clot colic. On examination, a mass is felt over the left loin and he has a left-sided varicocele.

☐ **2**   A 20-month-old baby boy is brought to the paediatric surgical clinic by his mother who gives a history of failure to thrive, fever and occasional blood in the nappy. On examination, a soft mass that does not cross the midline is palpable on the right side of the abdomen.

☐ **3**   A 35-year-old man of Asian origin presents with evening rise of temperature, weight loss, increased urinary frequency and painful micturition. Urine investigation reveals a sterile pyuria.

☐ **4**   A 67-year-old smoker presents with a 5-month history of painless haematuria, increased frequency of micturition and loss of weight. He worked in the dye industry before his retirement.

120 THEME: ACID–BASE BALANCE/STATUS

A   Acute renal failure
B   Flail chest
C   Pulmonary embolus
D   Pyloric stenosis

For each of the acid–base disturbance conditions given below, select the most likely diagnosis from the above list. Each option may be used once, more than once, or not at all.

☐ **1**   Hypocapnia

☐ **2**   Metabolic acidosis

☐ **3**   Metabolic alkalosis

121 THEME: ACID–BASE BALANCE

A   Metabolic acidosis   D   Respiratory acidosis
B   Metabolic alkalosis   E   Respiratory alkalosis
C   Normal pH

For each of the patients described below, select the most likely acid–base status from the list of options above. Each option may be used once, more than once, or not at all.

☐ **1**   A 70-year-old man with chronic obstructive pulmonary disease collapses on the ward after being admitted with an exacerbation of infection.

☐ **2**   A 65-year-old man admitted with epigastric pain, vomiting and jaundice. A serum amylase level of 2000 IU was recorded.

☐ **3**   A 41-year-old woman with shortness of breath and haemoptysis, and complaining of chest pain, was noted to have unilateral leg swelling 4–6 months after a right upper lobectomy for carcinoma of the lung.

122 THEME: ACID–BASE BALANCE

	pH	$Paco_2$	HCO_3^-
A	7.20	3.1	11
B	7.42	6.1	35
C	7.56	3.0	30

For each of the patients described below, select the most likely set of blood gas measurements from the list of options above. Each option may be used once, more than once, or not at all.

☐ 1 A 68-year-old woman with a history of abdominal pain with rebound tenderness and guarding for 72 hours. She exhibits signs of peritonitis and a WBC of 23×10^9/l.

☐ 2 A 45-year-old woman who had a total abdominal hysterectomy for fibroids is now complaining of shortness of breath 7 days after surgery. There is no history of haemoptysis or pleuritic chest pain.

☐ 3 A 75-year-old man had an uneventful abdominal aortic aneurysm (AAA) repair 10 days ago. He is known to smoke 30 cigarettes per day.

123 THEME: AUDIT

A Criterion
B Incident review
C Outcome
D Strategic

For each of the following situations select the most likely answer from the above list. Each option may be used once, more than once, or not at all.

☐ 1 Assessment of trauma patients who are brought into the Emergency Department unconscious and hypotensive to evaluate whether colloid fluids were given.

☐ 2 The use of emergency IVU.

ANSWERS

ANSWERS

1 CONSENT FOR SURGICAL TREATMENT

1 E – Yes, surgery can proceed
Surgery is needed for the preservation of life and can be performed despite the patient's inability to give consent. The patient's wife cannot give permission or stop her husband's operation. No adult can act as legal proxy for any other in the UK with regard to giving consent for surgical treatment.

2 A – Apply to make the child a ward of court
The surgeon can either respect the patient's wishes and not subject the child to an operation or can make an application for the child to be made a ward of court and proceed with appropriate surgical treatment. In this case surgical treatment is essential and almost all surgeons would do the latter.

3 E – Yes, surgery can proceed
The Mental Health Act does not allow for the compulsory treatment of any medical condition other than a mental disorder. The orthopaedic surgeon may, however, proceed with surgery for the patient's fractured femur if he or she and the patient's psychiatrist agree that it is the best form of management for her. It is good clinical practice to also obtain a second consultant's surgical opinion, confirming the need for operative treatment and to involve the relatives in the decision-making process where possible. Every clinician should make detailed entries in the patient's records and sign and date them.

4 B – No, surgery cannot proceed
No. Before the deterioration of this patient's condition he clearly refused to consent to operative treatment. Therefore, surgery cannot be performed even when he is unable to express his refusal for such a seemingly essential intervention.

2   DEATH AND THE LAW

1   A – Any medical practitioner
2   D – Medical practitioner who attended during previous 14 days
3   B – Coroner
4   E – Registrar of births and deaths

A doctor may issue a death certificate if he or she is a registered medical practitioner. In practice, this usually means where the doctor attended within 14 days of the death. Only the coroner is entitled to hold an inquest on any case that is reported to him/her.

3   DEATH CERTIFICATES

1   E – Report to the coroner
2   C – Issue a death certificate

Death should be referred to the coroner if:

> The cause of death is unknown.
> The deceased was not seen by the certifying doctor either after death or within 14 days before death.
> The death may be due to an accident.
> The death was unnatural, violent or suspicious.
> The death may be due to self-neglect or neglect by others (as in scenario 1).
> The death may be due to an abortion.
> The death may be a suicide.
> The death may be occupational/as a result of industrial disease.
> The death occurred during/after detention in police custody or prison.
> The death is during or within 24 hours of an operation/anaesthetic/invasive procedure

For scenario 1, it is common practice to telephone the coroner to get advice for death following an operation. However, according to the guidelines above, this is not strictly necessary.

4   CANCER THERAPY OPTIONS

1   D – Systemic chemotherapy
Prolonged remission, or even cure, can be achieved using systemic chemotherapy for recurrent non-Hodgkin's lymphoma.

2   C – Surgical resection
Isolated pulmonary metastasis from colorectal cancer (as occurs in 5% of patients) can be surgically removed with curative intent if the patient will tolerate a thoracotomy. It is only suitable if the primary tumour has been rigorously controlled and extrathoracic secondaries have been excluded.

3   C – Surgical resection
Residual anal squamous cell carcinoma post local radiotherapy is best treated by abdominoperineal resection with curative intent.

4   A – Hormonal manipulation
Metastatic prostatic carcinoma not involving bone is best treated by hormonal manipulation. If the bone is involved, radiotherapy is the treatment of choice, with or without internal fixation.

5   B – Radiotherapy and steroids
Multiple intracranial metastases are best treated with radiotherapy, whether over the whole brain or with stereotactic radiosurgery (gamma knife). Diffuse intracranial metastatic melanoma has an extremely poor prognosis. Short-term benefit may be achieved by radiotherapy with steroids; chemotherapy is of no benefit.

5   MALIGNANT MELANOMA

1   **C – Lentigo maligna melanoma**
2   **A – Acral lentiginous melanoma**
3   **C – Lentigo maligna melanoma**
4   **E – Superficial spreading melanoma**

Superficial spreading melanoma (65% of cases) is the commonest form of cutaneous malignant melanoma. Lentigo maligna is preceded by, or occurs within, a Hutchinson's melanotic freckle and is most commonly found on the face. Both of the above melanomas have a pronounced horizontal growth phase. Lentigo maligna melanoma and thin superficial spreading melanomas (< 0.76 mm) have a good prognosis. Acral lentiginous melanomas have a predilection for sites of thick epidermis such as the sole of the foot and have a poorer prognosis. Nodular melanomas have a pronounced vertical growth phase and hence a poor prognosis.

6   HISTOLOGICAL TUMOUR TYPES

1   **B – Neoplastic polyp**
2   **A – Hamartoma**
3   **A – Hamartoma**
4   **C – Neuroendocrine tumour**
5   **C – Neuroendocrine tumour**
6   **D – Gastrointestinal stromal tumour**
7   **C – Neuroendocrine tumour**

Hamartomas resemble tumours but they are not neoplastic. They result from a localised disorder of the relationships of normal tissues, leading to overproduction of one or more elements without the growth characteristics of tumours. Gastrointestinal stromal cell tumours arise from smooth muscle or Schwann cells. They have different grades of malignancy and spectrum of aggressiveness. They are relatively radioresistant and chemoresistant. Recently, studies have demonstrated expression of *c-kit*, a tyrosine kinase receptor. Chemotherapy in the form of an antibody to *c-kit*, called CD117 (Glivec (imantinib)) has been shown to be effective against this tumour (80% cases).

7 TUMOUR MARKERS

1 **C – β-hCG**
2 **B – α-fetoprotein**
3 **A – Acid phosphatase**
4 **D – Carcinoembryonic antigen (CEA)**
5 **E – Paraproteins**
Multiple myeloma is associated with the secretion of paraproteins, which may be seen on an electrophoretic strip. Light-chain protein (Bence Jones) is secreted into the urine in myeloma.

A proportion of colorectal carcinomas secrete carcinoembryonic antigen (CEA). CEA has a limited role in the follow-up of patients with colorectal cancer. Interpretation and intervention of late rises in CEA remains controversial.

Hepatomas may secrete α-fetoprotein, and teratomas β-hCG. Though not diagnostic, they have some role in screening investigation of tumours. They are useful for follow-up of recurrence.

Acid phosphatase is now an uncommonly used marker of prostatic cancer, as it has a low specificity. Prostatic specific antigen (PSA) is a much better tumour marker in terms of sensitivity and specificity.

8 CHEMOTHERAPY REGIMENS

1 **B – Colorectal carcinoma**
2 **A – Breast carcinoma**
3 **D – Testicular seminoma**
Several studies have now shown a limited survival benefit for Duke's C and Duke's B colorectal cancer using adjuvant treatment with combination 5-fluorouracil (5-FU) and folinic acid. Seminomas of the testis are sensitive to the combination of bleomycin, cisplatin and etoposide, and this has led to a marked improvement in survival rates in recent years. Adjuvant treatment for cancer of the breast using a combination of cyclophosphamide, methotrexate and 5-FU (CMF regimen) has been shown to prolong survival, especially in women who are node-positive and < 70 years. Doxorubicin (adriamycin) has been shown to improve survival for breast cancer and is replacing CMF in some centres.

Answers

9 TESTICULAR TUMOURS

1 C – Teratoma
2 B – Seminoma
3 C – Teratoma
4 C – Teratoma
5 A – Choriocarcinoma

Teratomas produce α-FP in about 70% of cases, secrete β-hCG in about 60% of cases, and secrete either α-FP or β-hCG in about 90% of cases.

Almost all choriocarcinomas secrete β-hCG, but they do not produce α-FP.

Less than 10% of seminomas secrete β-hCG, and very rarely produce α-FP.

10 HORMONE-SECRETING TUMOURS

1 B – α-fetoprotein
2 A – ACTH
3 C – Calcitonin
4 F – 5-hydroxytryptamine
5 D – Erythropoietin

α-Fetoprotein is secreted in high amounts by hepatocellular carcinomas (90%) and teratomas.

Bronchial carcinomas may secrete a variety of hormones including ACTH, cortisol, antidiuretic hormone (ADH) and parathormone.

Medullary thyroid carcinoma is known to secrete calcitonin (from parafollicular C cells), which can be used as a tumour marker.

Renal carcinoma may present with polycythaemia as part of a paraneoplastic syndrome. This is due to excess secretion of erythropoietin.

11 SKIN LESIONS

1 **F – S-100 positive on immunohistochemical staining**
2 **E – Palisading basal cells at the periphery of tumour islands**
3 **D – Keratin pearl formation**
4 **B – Intraepidermal (in situ) squamous carcinoma**
5 **A – Central keratin plug**
Basal cell carcinoma characteristically has palisading basal cells at the periphery of tumour islands.

Most cutaneous malignant melanomas stain S-100 positive using immunohistochemical techniques.

Squamous-cell carcinoma displays keratin pearl formation.

Bowen's disease is an in situ squamous cell carcinoma. Lesions appear as reddened, scaly, slightly raised plaques. Invasion occurs only after many years, typically 15–20 years.

A keratoacanthoma is a self-limiting, benign cutaneous tumour. A small red swelling grows quickly into a pale dome-shaped mass with a central keratin plug. These lesions regress spontaneously.

Paget's disease of the breast represents intraepithelial spread from an underlying ductal carcinoma.

12 LOCAL ANAESTHETIC AGENTS

1 **A – Amethocaine**
2 **B – Bupivacaine**
3 **D – Cocaine**
Amethocaine is an ester that rapidly diffuses into the conjunctiva. Cocaine is also an ester but causes sympathetic stimulation, and so is reserved for situations where vasoconstriction is required (eg nasal procedures).

All the other local anaesthetics are amides. Bupivacaine binds to the myocardium and has caused a number of deaths when used in Bier's blocks. Thus, it is now contraindicated for use in Bier's blocks. Prilocaine binds poorly to the myocardium and so is the best agent for intravenous regional anaesthesia.

13 OPERATIVE MANAGEMENT

1   **B – Carry on with surgery regardless**
2   **B – Carry on with surgery regardless**
3   **E – Wait 4 weeks**

Appendicitis in pregnancy may be difficult to diagnose due to upward displacement of the appendix and masking of guarding by the uterus. The later into the pregnancy, the greater is the mortality risk to the mother and fetus. A patient with acute appendicitis who is on the oral contraceptive pill should have an emergency operation. Neither pregnancy, nor taking the oral contraceptive pill is a contraindication to appendicectomy. The correct procedure for women on the oral contraceptive pill is to carry on with the surgery but take precautionary measures, such as thromboembolic deterrent stockings (TEDS), pneumatic calf compression and administration of heparin or low-molecular-weight heparins.

A patient requiring elective right inguinal hernia repair taking the oral contraceptive pill should have the surgery delayed, as the risk of potential complications (ie PE) would outweigh waiting for 1 month and then performing the surgery. During this 1-month delay, the patient should be advised to stop taking the oral contraceptive pill and to use other forms of contraception.

14 TUMOUR TYPE

1   **B – Lymphoma**
2   **D – Sarcoma**
3   **E – Squamous cell carcinoma**
4   **A – Adenocarcinoma**
5   **A – Adenocarcinoma**

Epstein–Barr virus infection may lead to Burkitt's lymphoma, which usually first appears in the jaw, and which shows a 'starry sky' appearance of a few macrophages in a sea of lymphoblasts on histology. Epstein–Barr virus is also responsible for nasopharyngeal carcinoma.

Muscle tumours arise from connective tissue, rather than epithelium. They are therefore sarcomas and not carcinomas. Striated muscle malignant tumours are therefore rhabdomyosarcomas. Malignant tumours arising from smooth muscle are leiomyosarcomas.

The human papillomavirus types 16 and 18 are responsible for CIN, and ultimately carcinoma of the cervix or anus. Of these 95% are squamous cell in origin, and 5% are adenocarcinomas.

Barrett's oesophagus arises as glandular dysplasia (from squamous to glandular epithelium), usually as a result of continued acid reflux.

Krukenberg tumours represent the transcoelomic spread of gastric carcinoma to the ovaries.

15 PARANEOPLASTIC SYNDROMES

1 **F – Thymoma**
2 **E – Renal carcinoma**
3 **C – Multiple myeloma**
4 **D – Pancreatic carcinoma**
Myasthenia gravis is seen with some thymic tumours.

Polycythaemia may arise from tumours of the kidney or cerebellum as a result of increased erythropoietin production.

Hypercalcaemia results from bone mobilisation from bony metastases and ectopic parathormone. It is most commonly seen in myeloma, breast and lung cancer.

Pancreatic carcinoma may lead to hyperglycaemia if enough β cells are destroyed – but this is rare.

Gout sometimes accompanies lymphoma.

Thrombophlebitis migrans is especially associated with lung and pancreatic cancer.

16 MODE OF TUMOUR SPREAD

1 **C – Lymphatic spread**
2 **B – Local invasion**
3 **C – Lymphatic spread**
4 **A – Blood-borne spread**
5 **D – Transcoelomic spread**

Seminomas of the testis and papillary thyroid carcinoma spread predominantly by the lymphatic route. Spread of testicular tumours follows their blood supply, and drainage is into the para-aortic lymph nodes. Remember that inguinal lymph nodes drain local skin, including the scrotum.

Cutaneous basal-cell carcinomas invade local structures and are hence termed 'rodent ulcers'. They rarely, if ever, spread to lymphatics or metastasise.

Follicular thyroid carcinomas spread predominantly by the bloodstream.

Ovarian carcinomas frequently spread transcoelomically.

17 ARTERIAL BLOOD GAS ANALYSIS/ACID–BASE BALANCE

1 B – Metabolic acidosis
The pH is low in scenario 1, representing a picture of acidosis. As the P_{CO_2} is reduced, this indicates that the cause is not respiratory. The bicarbonate is low, suggesting a metabolic acidosis.

2 D – Respiratory acidosis
In the second scenario, the pH is low, representing a picture of acidosis. The P_{CO_2} is raised, indicating a respiratory origin. The bicarbonate is normal so there has been no renal compensation. This picture may be seen in narcosis due to excess administration of opiates.

3 C – Metabolic alkalosis
The pH in the last case is high, so representing an alkalosis. The bicarbonate level too is very high, so indicating a metabolic origin. The P_{CO_2} is slightly high because of respiratory compensation. An example of this is seen in gastric outflow obstruction.

18 SHOCK

1 B – Fat embolism
Fat embolism occurs in patients with multiple closed fractures, but has been reported in those with other skeletal trauma and burns. Fat embolism causes a pyrexia, tachycardia, shortness of breath, confusion and petechial haemorrhages, especially on the chest and conjunctivae.

2 D – Thromboembolism
Post-operative day 7 is the characteristic time for a thromboembolism.

3 C – Hypovolaemic shock
Scenario 3 describes a leaking abdominal aortic aneurysm (AAA). Management involves immediate transfer to the operating theatre for laparotomy and emergency grafting of his AAA.

19 5-YEAR SURVIVAL RATES OF TUMOURS

1 C – > 95%
2 G – 90–95%
3 D – 5–10%
4 A – < 5%
5 B – 25%
6 F – 70–75%

The overall 5-year survival rates of patients with carcinoid tumours depend on the site of the primary. Those of the appendix have an approximate 98% 5-year survival; those of the rectum an 85% survival; and those of the small bowel have the lowest survival rate.

The 5-year survival rates (Duke's A, B and C rectal cancers) have improved from the easily memorised '90%, 60%, and 30%', respectively, to 92% (A), 71% (B), 40% (C1) and 26% (C2).

Oesophageal and pancreatic cancers have a grave prognosis, and surgical cure is uncommon.

Metastatic prostatic cancer can frequently be temporarily controlled by hormonal treatment.

20 LYMPH NODES

1   C – Para-aortic
2   B – External iliac
3   D – Superficial inguinal
4   C – Para-aortic

Lymphatics from the testicles run with the arteries and drain into the aortic nodes. Lymphatic spread of tumour from the cervix occurs in 40% of women, with preferential spread to the external iliac, internal iliac and obturator nodes. Drainage from the anal canal is to the internal iliac nodes from the upper part and to the superficial inguinal nodes from the lower part. Lymphatic vessels from the rectum pass directly to the aortic nodes.

21 TYPES OF ULCERATION

1   C – Marjolin's ulcer
2   B – Cushing's ulcer
3   A – Curling's ulcer
4   E – Pyoderma gangrenosum

Marjolin's ulcers are squamous cell carcinomas (SCCs) that develop in long-standing chronic venous ulcers. Gastroduodenal stress ulcers follow major trauma or sepsis. The pathophysiology is unclear, but is thought to relate to relative mucosal ischaemia, lack of oral alimentation and altered gastric mucous barrier function. Specific forms of gastroduodenal stress ulceration include: Cushing's ulcer, which follows severe head injury; and Curling's ulcer, which follows major burns. Pyoderma gangrenosum occurs in inflammatory bowel disease, and is more common in ulcerative colitis than Crohn's disease.

22 PATHOLOGIES OF THE FEMORO-INGUINAL REGION

1   D – Strangulated femoral hernia
2   J – Saphena varix
3   A – Psoas abscess
4   F – False aneurysm of the femoral artery

Femoral hernia is due to the protrusion of extra-peritoneal tissue and some abdominal contents through the femoral canal. It is more common in females (two and a half times) as the inguinal ligament makes a wider angle with the pubis. Femoral canal is bounded supero-anteriorly by the inguinal ligament, infero-posteriorly by the pubic ramus and pectineus muscle, medially by lacunar ligament and laterally by the femoral vein. Femoral hernia is differentiated from inguinal hernia as it lies lateral and inferior to pubic tubercle, while the inguinal hernia lies medial and above the pubic tubercle. Strangulated hernia is characterised by pain, irreducibility, and absent cough impulse. Necrosis of the involved viscus ensues with progressive loss of blood supply and this may lead to local, and then systemic sepsis, if untreated. The patients may present with general ill-health, vomiting and constipation. Associated pyrexia may be present if the infection becomes systemic.

Saphena varix is a saccular enlargement of the vein, usually seen at the proximal part of the long saphenous venous system. This is commonly seen in patients with varicose veins. The patients present with a swelling over the medial part of the upper thigh (where the long saphenous vein enters the femoral vein piercing the cribriform fascia) and the swelling often has a blue tinge. It disappears on lying down due to the emptying of the vein into the deeper system (femoral vein). There might be a palpable thrill when the patient coughs and an impulse is felt over the varix when the vein is tapped from below (Schwart's test).

Psoas abscess is usually due to a cold abscess tracking down towards the inguinal region from the spine along the psoas muscle. This is usually due to tuberculosis affecting the spine (Pott's disease). The abscess is usually fluctuant, painless and not warm (hence the name cold abscess which is characteristic of tuberculosis). Often there may be cross fluctuation (above the inguinal ligament) due to an associated iliac abscess. The diagnosis is made from the history and clinical examination. It can be confirmed either by radiograph, ultrasound or CT scanning of the spine. Associated organ involvement should be actively looked for such as lung involvement, for example.

False aneurysm of the femoral artery occurs as a result of laceration or injury to the arterial wall (usually tunica adventitia). The injury leads to local haematoma which becomes contained in the surrounding normal tissue. There is often a history of considerable primary haemorrhage from the wound which usually settles with sustained pressure. This is common with IV drug abusers as they may accidentally puncture the femoral artery when attempting to inject the drug into the adjacent femoral vein as the artery and the vein lies in close proximity in the femoral triangle. Distal pulsation in the affected limb is usually maintained. There may be local bruit over the involved arterial region and the appearance of the expansile pulsation in the region usually clinches the diagnosis.

23 ABDOMINAL DISEASE

1 G – Mesenteric ischaemia
The finding of atrial fibrillation in a patient with sudden-onset abdominal pain must raise the possibility of an embolic event. Embolism accounts for 25–30% of patients with mesenteric ischaemia. It is notoriously difficult to diagnose and the passage of blood per rectum is relatively rare.

2 D – Crohn's disease
A longer history of diarrhoea and vomiting over several months, together with a vague right iliac fossa mass and established microcytic anaemia, is more suggestive of Crohn's disease because of iron loss from haemorrhage. A macrocytic anaemia may also be seen as a result of vitamin B12 malabsorption due to terminal ileitis.

3 A – Appendix mass
An appendix mass forms when an inflamed appendix perforates locally and pus is prevented from spreading throughout the peritoneal cavity by adherent omentum and small bowel. The patient has a history suggesting appendicitis, and occasionally a tender mass may be felt in the right iliac fossa.

24 INVESTIGATIONS FOR ABDOMINAL PAIN

1 A – CT abdomen
The most likely diagnosis for the first patient is appendicitis. FBC measurement is useful in lending support to the diagnosis, in that it may show a neutrophilia, but a normal reading should not affect management. CT of the abdomen has been used more recently to diagnose appendicitis.

2 C – Erect chest X-ray
Patient 2 has a good history for perforation of a viscus, probably a peptic ulcer – she is on several ulcer-promoting medications. An erect chest X-ray (CXR) should be performed after the patient has been upright for several minutes to look for free gas under the diaphragm.

3 E – Mesenteric angiography
While an FBC is important in patient 3 it will not lead to diagnosing the cause of the problem. A mesenteric angiogram is useful if the patient is bleeding at a rate of > 1 ml/min.

4 F – Supine abdominal X-ray
Patient 4 may be developing acute intestinal obstruction. This is more likely after operations on the lower part of the abdomen. A supine abdominal X-ray will aim to show any dilated loops.

25 ABDOMINAL PAIN INVESTIGATIONS – DIAGNOSTIC

1 H – Serum amylase
Serum amylase estimation would be the most appropriate investigation for the first clinical case scenario, as the most likely diagnosis is pancreatitis. A subsequent CT may be needed if findings are equivocal.

2 D – Barium meal – small bowel follow-through
The history of the young man is suggestive of Crohn's disease and a barium meal with small bowel follow-through would be the most appropriate investigation.

3 F – Erect chest X-ray
The third patient is most likely to have a perforated peptic ulcer as evidenced by the epigastric pain, shallow respirations and tachycardia. This would be suspected because of oral steroid and non-steroidal intake. An erect chest X-ray would be the most appropriate investigation.

4   G – FBC
The most appropriate investigation in the fourth patient would be a full blood count as the rectal bleeding has led her to become tachycardic and hypotensive. If profuse bleeding continues, she will require a mesenteric angiogram and possible embolisation of the bleeding vessel.

26   INVESTIGATIONS OF THE GASTROINTESTINAL TRACT

1   A – Colonoscopy
In the first case, one would suspect or need to exclude a colonic tumour, polyp or angiodysplasia. Thus, a colonoscopy would be the most appropriate investigation. Some would advocate an initial colonoscopy, as this patient is in the at-risk age group for developing colonic polyps/tumour.

2   A – Colonoscopy
The second case represents a patient with a sigmoid volvulus, and the most appropriate investigation here would be a colonoscopy to decompress the volvulus. A rigid sigmoidoscopy may be done in the Emergency Department to achieve the same effect.

27   PANCREATITIS

1   B – Acute-on-chronic pancreatitis
The 43-year-old alcoholic with pain radiating to his back relieved by leaning forward is most likely to have chronic pancreatitis. A very similar picture can be seen with carcinoma of the head of the pancreas, but the one discriminating feature is that pain is constant and persistent in carcinoma. Moreover, the peak incidence of pancreatic adenocarcinoma is 60–80 years of age.

2   E – Pancreatic pseudocyst
A patient who is alcoholic with a history of chronic pancreatitis and a palpable abdominal mass suggests a pancreatic pseudocyst. This can be easily diagnosed by ultrasound or CT scan.

3   A – Acute pancreatitis
This final clinical case is typical of acute pancreatitis with a history of sudden onset of pain, vomiting and an increased serum amylase level.

28 CHOLECYSTECTOMY

1 D – ERCP
An ERCP is a useful method of removing stones from the common bile duct to relieve jaundice. It is associated with a 1% risk of pancreatitis and a 0.1% risk of mortality.

2 B – Elective cholecystectomy
If patients are fit enough and are symptomatic from gallstones, then a cholecystectomy should be performed. Nearly 90% of all cholecystectomies are performed laparoscopically in the UK.

29 PANCREATIC TUMOUR

1 C – Insulinoma
Insulinomas produce episodes of hypoglycaemia leading to altered behaviour and disturbances of consciousness. Characteristically, the patient feels well between episodes. It is a difficult diagnosis to make unless there is a degree of clinical suspicion.

2 E – Zollinger–Ellison syndrome
In the second case, the patient has MEN-1. The hypercalcaemia arises from hyperparathyroidism. He also has Zollinger–Ellison syndrome, which causes markedly raised levels of gastrin and gastric acid hypersecretion. This leads to severe ulceration not only in the stomach and duodenum but also the jejunum.

30 SIDE-EFFECTS OF TREATMENT FOR INFLAMMATORY BOWEL DISEASE

1 D – Metronidazole
2 E – Sulfasalazine
3 B – Corticosteroids
4 B – Corticosteroids
5 C – Methotrexate
6 C – Methotrexate

As well as nausea and vomiting, metronidazole may cause peripheral neuropathy, convulsions, headaches and hepatitis. Metronidazole is associated with irreversible peripheral neuropathy and does not appear to be related to the dose or length of time of ingestion.

Hepatic fibrosis and pneumonitis from methotrexate use is related to the total dose given. Other adverse effects include: myelosuppression, nausea and vomiting, stomatitis, diarrhoea, osteoporosis, renal dysfunction, acute vasculitis (if high doses used) and seizures (especially after intrathecal use).

Osteoporosis and cataracts are well-known complications of corticosteroids. Susceptibility to infection, Cushingoid appearance, central obesity, buffalo hump, moon facies, diabetes, hypertension, peptic ulceration, thin and easily bruised skin, striae, mental changes and proximal myopathy are associated side-effects.

31 SURGICAL INVESTIGATIONS

1 G **B** – Gastrografin enema
2 B – Abdominal ultrasound
3 A – Abdominal and pelvic CT scan
4 H **G** – Small bowel follow-through
5 **G** – Gastrografin enema

An acutely obstructing large bowel cancer is best assessed with a gastrografin (water soluble) enema. This is because use of barium in the enema may result in a severe peritonitis if it leaks through a bowel perforation into the peritoneum. Colonoscopy is associated with an increased risk of perforation.

A barium enema clearly defines the presence and extent of colonic diverticular disease, but a CT scan would identify an abscess associated with diverticular disease.

Mesenteric fat stranding and localised inflammatory changes would be seen with a CT scan. Acute and chronic gallbladder pathology is best seen on ultrasound.

Small bowel pathology is currently not well imaged by other forms of investigation other than follow-through contrast examinations. More recently, capsule endoscopy has been shown to be useful in diagnosis of bleeding in the small bowel.

Early colonic anastomotic leaks are best assessed using gastrografin enemas or CT.

32 SURGICAL INVESTIGATIONS

1 **A – Abdominal CT scan**
2 **G – Small bowel follow-through**
3 **C – Barium enema (double contrast)**
4 **A – Abdominal CT scan**
No technique is certain to reveal a colovesical fistula, but cystoscopy and barium enema are the two most likely investigations to help (one may see air in the bladder). X-ray of spun urine following a barium enema may also reveal barium radio-opacity. Pancreatic necrosis is not well visualised on ultrasound. Dynamic CT scans will usually demonstrate non-perfused pancreatic tissue.

33 ABDOMINAL DISEASE

1 **C – Familial adenomatous polyposis**
2 **E – Ulcerative colitis**
3 **A – Crohn's disease**
4 **A – Crohn's disease**
5 **E – Ulcerative colitis**
6 **B – Diverticular disease**
Desmoid tumours are benign proliferations of well-differentiated fibroblasts. Typically they occur in the lower rectus sheath and infiltrate the surrounding tissues. They are associated with intestinal tumours and Gardner's syndrome (multiple osteomas and familial adenomatous polyposis).

Enteroenteric fistulas are more likely to complicate Crohn's disease than diverticular disease. Diverticular disease accounts for approximately half of all colovesical fistulas, and Crohn's disease comprises only about 15–20%.

Pyoderma gangrenosum, ankylosing spondylitis and toxic megacolon are more common in ulcerative colitis than in Crohn's disease. Anal pathology is much more prevalent in Crohn's disease.

34 HERNIAS

1 D – Lumbar hernia
2 C – Gluteal hernia
3 F – Perineal hernia
4 H – Spigelian hernia

Lumbar hernias occur through either the inferior lumbar triangle of Petit (bounded by the iliac crest, the posterior edge of the external oblique and the anterior edge of the latissimus dorsi) or the superior lumbar space (bounded by the 12th rib, the lower border of the serratus posterior inferior as well as the anterior border of the sacrospinalis and the internal oblique).

A perineal hernia is seen as a rare complication of abdominoperineal (A-P) resection, and develops through a non-healing perineal wound.

35 POLYPS

1 A – Inflammatory polyps
2 C – Peutz–Jeghers polyps
3 E – Villous adenomatous polyps
4 E – Villous adenomatous polyps
5 D – Tubular adenomatous polyps

Villous adenomas of the rectum frequently present with the passage of bright-red blood and mucus per rectum. If villous adenomas are large, mucus secretion is significant and hypokalaemia may occur. Villous adenomas have the greatest malignant potential of all colorectal polyps. Peutz–Jeghers polyps have no malignant potential themselves, but are associated with an increased risk of other malignant gut polyps.

Metaplastic polyps are also known as hyperplastic polyps. They are symptomless, occurring throughout the large bowel and are the most common type of polyp found in the rectum. They are thought not to undergo dysplastic or neoplastic change. Inflammatory polyps have no malignant potential.

36 GASTROINTESTINAL HAEMORRHAGE

1 E – Oesophagogastroduodenoscopy
Any patient who attends the Emergency Department with a massive fresh bleed per rectum that causes haemodynamic compromise should undergo an oesophagogastroduodenoscopy to exclude a bleeding peptic ulcer. Only after this has been excluded should one proceed with lower GI investigations.

2 A – Colonoscopy
In the second case, the elderly man is not in shock and the nature of the bleeding is suggestive of a lower GI cause, eg diverticular disease or colonic carcinoma. In this instance a colonoscopy would probably be the best first-line investigation.

3 A – Colonoscopy
In the third case, the young man who presents to the clinic with no local cause for the rectal bleeding should undergo a colonoscopy to exclude a polyp. This investigation is preferable to a barium enema as it may be therapeutic as well as diagnostic and has a higher specificity and sensitivity. CT colonography for the screening of polyps and colonic cancer is currently undergoing evaluation.

37 HERNIAS

1 C – Pantaloon hernia
2 B – Maydl's hernia
3 E – Sliding hernia
4 D – Richter's hernia
5 A – Littré's hernia

In a sliding hernia the posterior wall of the hernial sac is formed by a herniating viscus. This is usually sigmoid colon or bladder. During repair, particular care is required not to injure the herniated viscus, which can be seen when examining inside the opened sac.

38 JAUNDICE

1 D – Duodenal carcinoma
Patient 1 has FAP. Such patients have adenomas in the colon and duodenum. The commonest extraintestinal manifestation of FAP is a duodenal carcinoma. Duodenal carcinoma should be suspected in a patient with FAP who becomes jaundiced. The tumour here appears to be causing extrahepatic biliary obstruction.

2 A – Acute cholangitis
Patient 2 exhibits altered features of Charcot's triad: fever, pain and rigors. Cholangitis is usually the result of a stone in the common bile duct.

3 B – Biliary colic
Patient 3 is most likely to have biliary colic, as this does not usually cause jaundice.

39 JAUNDICE

1 C – Empyema of the gallbladder
A palpable right upper quadrant mass, fever and the feeling of being generally unwell would point to an empyema of the gallbladder.

2 B – Common bile-duct stone
Obstructive jaundice 48 hours after open cholecystectomy is most likely the result of a common bile duct (CBD) calculus, which was missed at the time of surgery. This could have been avoided if a pre-operative ultrasound had shown dilatation of the CBD stones would have been visualised and removed by pre-operative ERCP.

Alternatively, during an open cholecystectomy, an intraoperative cholangiogram can be performed to visualise stones in the CBD. The CBD can then be opened, the stones removed and a T-tube left in situ.

3 E – Mucocele of the gallbladder
A stone in Hartmann's pouch causing right quadrant upper pain is most likely to lead to a mucocele.

40 PANCREATIC TUMOURS

1 B – Glucagonoma
Glucagonomas are rare, but present with long-standing eczematous rash (usually > 1 year), glossitis, stomatitis, diabetes and wasting.

2 C – Insulinoma
Clinical features of insulinomas include disturbances of consciousness and 'odd' behaviour; in fact almost any neurological or psychiatric syndrome can be mimicked. Conversation and movement may be restricted during attacks, but the patient feels normal between attacks. This behaviour is part of the MEN-1 syndrome.

Glucagonomas and insulinomas should be treated surgically because of the malignant potential of these tumours.

41 JAUNDICE

1 B – Post-hepatic jaundice
2 A – Hepatic jaundice
3 B – Post-hepatic jaundice
4 B – Post-hepatic jaundice
Pre-hepatic jaundice is associated with the presence of (urinary) urobilinogen and the absence of urinary bilirubin. Causes include recent blood transfusion and a family history of haemolytic syndromes.

Hepatic jaundice may be conjugated or unconjugated, and is associated with a history of recent foreign travel, alcohol or drug abuse, ingestion of hepatotoxic drugs (halothane, chlorpromazine) or liver tumours.

Post-hepatic jaundice is associated with bilirubin in the urine, a positive Courvoisier's sign (extrahepatic duct obstruction), pruritus, a history of fever, jaundice and rigors (Charcot's triad – due to ascending cholangitis) and a history of dark urine and pale stools.

42 RECTAL BLEEDING

1   **A – Crohn's disease**
2   **E – Meckel's diverticulum**
3   **H – Solitary juvenile polyp**
4   **B – Familial adenomatous polyposis**
5   **F – Mid-gut volvulus**
Rectal bleeding is a common symptom throughout childhood.

Crohn's disease may present in many ways but is frequently associated with weight loss or linear growth failure in children.

Meckel's diverticulum may present with acute GI haemorrhage leading to the typical brick-red coloured stool. Ulceration is caused by the ectopic gastric mucosa within the Meckel's diverticulum and may also cause lower abdominal pain.

Solitary juvenile polyps are a relatively common cause of painless rectal bleeding. Occasionally, juvenile polyps may be multiple.

Familial adenomatous polyposis should be suspected in children presenting with rectal bleeding when there is a family history of early colorectal carcinoma in immediate family members. The polyps generally develop after puberty.

Mid-gut volvulus is frequently preceded by a history of intermittent colicky abdominal pain with or without bile-stained vomiting – usually from the age of 3 months. This diagnosis should always be considered in a child with bile-stained vomiting and rectal bleeding.

43 ABDOMINAL PAIN

1   C – Renal adenocarcinoma
The presentation of the first patient is typically that of renal carcinoma; however, this triad of symptoms and signs only occurs in 30% of cases.

2   B – Pelviureteric obstruction
Loin pain in the patient who drinks four cups of coffee before work is most likely to be the result of pelviureteric obstruction. Symptoms of ureteric obstruction in adults usually occur after a fluid overload.

3   A – Leaking abdominal aortic aneurysm
Any male patient above the age of 55 years who presents with back pain should be suspected of having a leaking abdominal aortic aneurysm (AAA) until proven otherwise, as AAAs are more common in this age group than urinary stones.

44 LOIN PAIN

1   D – Pyelonephritis
One would suspect pyelonephritis in a male patient with loin pain, pyrexia and tachycardia.

2   G – Urinary calculi
In an 18-year-old man with right iliac fossa pain and microscopic haematuria, appendicitis or a urinary calculus should be suspected. With a perforated appendicitis, however, the patient lies still, unlike the writhing around with the pain of ureteric colic.

3   D – Pyelonephritis
Here the most likely diagnosis is pyelonephritis in view of the bilateral reflux, dysuria, malaise and fever.

45 SCROTAL SWELLINGS

1   **G – Varicocele**
2   **E – Testicular tumour**
3   **D – Inguinoscrotal hernia**
4   **C – Hydrocele**

A varicocele is often referred to as the sensation of a 'bag of worms' in the scrotum. The varicosities are more prominent when the patient is standing, and they disappear or decrease in size when the patient lies down.

An indirect inguinal hernia is more likely to occur on the right, as the right testis descends later. However, 98% of varicoceles occur on the left. The reasons for this are:
(1)   the left testicular vein forms a greater angle with the left renal vein;
(2)   the left renal vein is crossed and may be compressed by the pelvic colon;
(3)   the left testicular vein is longer than the right ; and
(4)   the terminal valve is frequently absent in the left testicular vein.

The history of onset of testicular tumour is varied, but is often associated with the onset of sudden pain. One should always suspect a testicular tumour if an irregular testis is ever felt, and an urgent ultrasound is required.

A painless, long-standing swelling that transilluminates within the scrotum is most likely to be a hydrocele. A hydrocele of the cord will be separate from the testis.

46 JAUNDICE

1 **B – Post-hepatic jaundice**
2 **A – Hepatic jaundice**
3 **C – Pre-hepatic jaundice**
4 **A – Hepatic jaundice**
5 **A – Hepatic jaundice**
6 **A – Hepatic jaundice**
7 **C – Pre-hepatic jaundice**
8 **B – Post-hepatic jaundice**
9 **A – Hepatic jaundice**
10 **C – Pre-hepatic jaundice**

Jaundice (icterus) is the yellow pigmentation of skin, sclera and mucosa due to a raised plasma bilirubin (> 35 mmol/l). Pruritus is the result of bile-salt deposition in the skin.

Pre-hepatic jaundice is associated with haemolytic anaemia and familial non-haemolytic hyperbilirubinaemia, such as in Gilbert's and Rotor's syndromes.

Hepatic causes include: acute viral or drug-induced (halothane, chlorpromazine) hepatitis; other hepatoxic substances (alcohol, carbon tetrachloride); cirrhosis, chronic active hepatitis; hepatic tumours, hydatid disease and liver abscesses.

Post-hepatic causes include: porta hepatis lymph nodes, sclerosing cholangitis, biliary atresia, bile duct carcinoma, pancreatic carcinoma and choledocholithiasis.

47 COLORECTAL SURGERY

1   A – Abdominoperineal resection
The first case is of a man with a recurrence of his anal carcinoma. He has undergone chemoradiotherapy which has failed. The only treatment for continued bleeding is surgery in the form of an abdominoperineal resection.

2   H – Subtotal colectomy
The second case is of a young woman with a flare-up of ulcerative colitis, failed medical treatment and development of a toxic megacolon. The surgical option now is a subtotal colectomy with ileostomy, as she is at imminent risk of perforation. The rectum is not excised, as this would increase the length of surgery and increase her morbidity. In addition, as she is young the possibility of a future ileoanal pouch should be left open to her.

3   C – Hartmann's procedure
The third case is of a probable perforated sigmoid carcinoma and single metastasis to the liver. The carcinoma should be resected. A primary anastomosis in the presence of gross faecal contamination would be unwise. However, purulent peritonitis is itself not an absolute contraindication to a primary anastomosis. This procedure should only be performed by an experienced surgeon and the majority would cover with a loop ileostomy.

48 MEDIASTINAL CONDITIONS

1   B – Aortic dissection
Aortic dissection produces tearing chest and back pain together with neurological deficits from spinal cord and cerebral ischaemia.

2   C – Carcinoma of the oesophagus
Oesophageal carcinoma is more common in elderly people and presents in advanced stages with progressive dysphagia.

3   D – Mallory–Weiss tear
A Mallory–Weiss tear produces a linear mucosal tear in the lower oesophagus close to the gastro-oesophageal junction, which results in haematemesis and later melaena.

Achalasia is the failure of the lower oesophageal sphincter to relax, with abnormal oesophageal peristalsis. It does not cause an anaemia unless there is malignant change.

49 MEDIASTINAL MASSES

1 **A – Anterior mediastinum**
2 **C – Posterior mediastinum**
3 **D – Superior mediastinum**
4 **A – Anterior mediastinum**
5 **B – Middle mediastinum**
The locations of mediastinal masses include:
Anterior mediastinum: thymic lesions, lymphoma, germ-cell tumours, pleuropericardial cysts, lymph node enlargement

Middle mediastinum: lymph node enlargement, bronchogenic cysts, enterogenic cysts

Posterior mediastinum: neural tumours, thoracic meningocele, oesophageal tumours, aortic aneurysms, paragangliomas

Superior mediastinum: thyroid masses, lymph node enlargement, oesophageal tumours, aortic aneurysms, parathyroid lesions

50 HEART MURMURS

1 **A – Continuous systolic murmur**
2 **E – Split second heart sound**
3 **B – Early diastolic murmur**
A ventricular septal defect will produce a continuous systolic murmur – pansystolic murmur, whereas an atrial septal defect will produce a wide and fixed splitting of the second heart sound.

A patient with aortic regurgitation has an early diastolic murmur.

51 CHEST INJURY

1 C – Pericardial injury
Scenario 1 is likely to be the result of a cardiac tamponade. Signs indicating this include a weak pulse, raised JVP, hypotension and tachycardia. The only other condition that may cause similar signs is a tension pneumothorax. However, the patient has a normal chest film which makes this unlikely.

2 D – Pneumothorax
The patient in scenario 2 is likely to have a pneumothorax as he has absent breath sounds, is dyspnoeic and drowsy as a result of hypoxia.

52 CARDIAC PHYSIOLOGY

1 B – HR, 50; SV, 140; PP, 50
2 F – HR, 200; SV, 35; PP, 50
3 C – HR, 100; SV, 70; PP, 70
Marathon runners have a high stroke volume and a resultant bradycardia. The resting cardiac output is approximately 6 litres/min.

Uncontrolled hyperthyroidism leads to a tachycardia and the most common arrhythmia is atrial fibrillation. It has no effect on the pulse pressure (PP). The cardiac output in these cases may be elevated.

53 DYSPNOEA

1 C – Left tension pneumothorax
The patient here has signs of a tension pneumothorax. No tracheal deviation is seen in cardiac tamponade.

2 D – Pulmonary embolus
Here, the characteristic ECG changes seen in pulmonary embolus are: S1, Q3, T3.

3 B – Left haemothorax
Dullness to percussion is indicative of fluid in the pleural space, hence the most appropriate answer here is a haemothorax.

54 MULTIPLE ENDOCRINE NEOPLASIA SYNDROMES

1   C – MEN IIB
2   A – MEN I
3   C – MEN IIB
4   A – MEN I

The multiple endocrine neoplasia syndromes (MEN) are inherited in an autosomal dominant manner or they may occur as new mutations. MEN I consists of pituitary, pancreatic islet cell and parathyroid adenomas or hyperplasia. Patients with MEN IIA and IIB develop phaeochromocytomas and medullary thyroid carcinomas. In addition, those with MEN IIA develop parathyroid hyperplasia, but are phenotypically normal; however, those with MEN IIB tend to be Marfanoid and develop submucosal neuromas.

55 UPPER ABDOMINAL PAIN

1   G – Pancreatitis

The diagnosis in this case would most likely be pancreatitis. The hypotension and tachycardia could suggest a visceral perforation or bleeding, but the most likely diagnosis would be pancreatitis with the history of steroids and back pain. Bruising in the flanks implies retroperitoneal bleeding. This is a feature of both pancreatitis and leaking aortic aneurysm, but in this age group with the history of steroid ingestion, the diagnosis of the former appears more likely.

2   D – Cholecystitis

Epigastric discomfort is a feature of both gallbladder and peptic ulcer disease. However, the presence of a pyrexia and raised WBC makes the former more likely, especially with the history of fatty food intolerance. Biliary colic does not cause a pyrexia or an elevated WBC.

3   I – Perforated duodenal ulcer

The presence of resonance over the liver suggests free intraperitoneal air. The most likely source of this from the above list is a perforated duodenal ulcer. Perforated gastric ulcer is another plausible option but its incidence is much lower.

56 RIGHT ILIAC FOSSA PAIN

1 H – Ureteric stone
There are no features here of peritonism. A patient with ureteric colic would typically pace around when they had the pain. A patient with peritonitis caused by a ruptured viscus would be lying still.

2 G – Terminal ileal Crohn's disease
The history here could be one of either Crohn's disease or irritable bowel syndrome. However, the weight loss would be more consistent with Crohn's disease. It should be noted that Crohn's or any inflammatory bowel problems pathology, including diverticular disease, can produce symptoms of functional bowel disorders: increased stool frequency, abdominal pain relieved by defaecation and faecal urgency.

57 TREATMENTS FOR ANAL PAIN

1 H – Solitary rectal ulcer syndrome
Solitary rectal ulcer syndrome is a relatively common cause of bright red rectal bleeding. It classically produces an ulcer on the anterior wall of the rectum, but may also have a polypoid appearance. The aetiology of the condition is incompletely understood but is thought to be a combination of internal intussusception/anterior wall prolapse and increased intrarectal pressure. The resultant symptoms are that of rectal evacuatory difficulty. Surgical treatment (abdominal rectopexy) is often unsatisfactory and the first line management is biofeedback.

2 G – Radiation proctitis
Radiation proctitis following treatment for cervical or prostatic cancer is a troublesome condition that is difficult to treat. Topical application of 4% formalin can help the bleeding. Other options include Nd: YAG laser, and surgery in the form of a coloanal sleeve anastamosis.

3 C – Low subcutaneous anal fistula (below the dentate line)

Treatment of anal fistula is complex when the tract extends high to involve a considerable portion of the external anal sphincter. The danger of laying open too much external anal sphincter is to render the patient incontinent. The difficulty in decision-making lies in estimating the 'safe' amount of sphincter to divide and thus how much sphincter is left behind. The decision varies according to the sex of the patient, the presence of sphincter defects, colonic and rectal function and also the patient. A low anal fistula, below the dentate line is usually safe to lay open; however, if there is concern regarding continence a seton (suture material: ethibond, nylon, silastic slings have all been used) can be placed through the tract to allow drainage and reassessment of treatment options.

4 B – Fissure in ano

Diltiazem is a calcium antagonist that reduces the resting pressure of the internal anal sphincter muscle (smooth muscle). Trials have shown this to be an effective treatment for acute and chronic anal fissures (65% healing rates).

5 B – Fissure in ano

Botulinum toxin has also been demonstrated to be an effective treatment for chronic anal fissure (73% efficacy). The precise mechanism of action is unclear, but reduced myogenic tone and contractile response to sympathetic stimulation by directly acting on its smooth muscle or indirectly on the nerves through inhibition of acetylcholine release are possibilities.

58 ABDOMINAL SYSTEM INVESTIGATIONS

1 B – Colonoscopy

Screening of colonic cancer in patients with a positive family history should be performed with colonoscopy as the whole colon must be visualised. The use of computed tomography (CT) colonography and magnetic resonance (MR) colonography for screening and primary detection of colorectal cancers is the subject of ongoing research.

2 C – CT

The problem here is the age of the patient and whether they would be able to tolerate a colonoscopy or barium enema investigation. It is common practice in many centres to use CT to identify a primary colorectal cancer in the over 80-year age group.

3   F – Flexible sigmoidoscopy
Bright red rectal bleeding in a young patient with no change in bowel habit can be suitably investigated with flexible sigmoidoscopy, as it is most likely that the source is located in the left colon.

4   B – Colonoscopy
Angiodysplasia of the colon is most commonly located in the ascending colon and caecum and is therefore best visualised by colonoscopy. Mesenteric angiography can also be used to demonstrate this vascular malformation. The malformations consist of dilated tortuous submucosal veins that may be replaced by massive dilated vessels in severe cases.

59   ABDOMINAL SYSTEM INVESTIGATIONS

1   G – MRI
Tissue invasion within the pelvis by rectal cancer is best assessed with MRI as this modality gives the best contrast resolution. MRI can identify whether the fascial envelope in which the rectum lies has been breached, or has a margin which may be threatened with tumour during surgical resection. With this technique, MRI can predict if neoadjuvant chemo-radiotherapy needs to be given.

2   B – CT
Hepatic metastases can be visualised by both MRI and CT. CT has better spatial resolution whereas MRI has superior contrast resolution.

3   C – Endoanal ultrasound
The most suitable investigation here would be an endoanal ultrasound to visualise the internal and external anal sphincters. Other investigations that need to be requested in such a patient would be anorectal manometry (to measure resting and squeeze anal pressures) and rectal sensory thresholds.

60 TIMING OF SURGICAL PROCEDURES

1   A – Urgent operation within next 12–24 hours
This lady has severe acute cholecystitis, which is not responding to antibiotics. The concern here is a possible empyema or gangrenous cholecystitis. Following urgent resuscitation, an emergency chole-cystectomy should be performed. This may be done laparoscopically or by open operation depending on the experience and skill of the operating surgeon. 'Hot' gallbladders, ie within the first 72 hours can be relatively easy to remove as the tissue oedema aids the dissection. However, if there have been recurrent episodes of inflammation or if the initial episode has been longer than 5 days, then surgery may be very difficult and a delay in operation should be considered.

2   D – Wait 6 weeks and operate
An appendix abscess can be treated conservatively with intravenous antibiotics as long as the patient responds to treatment. Indications for surgery are a persistent pyrexia, tachycardia and generalised peritonitis. The optimal time for an interval appendicectomy is debatable, but 6 weeks is a reasonable time period.

3   C – Wait 6 months and operate
The management of a post-operative enterocutaneous fistula is based initially on control of sepsis, nutrition (enteral or parenteral) and wound management. Subsequent anatomical mapping of the fistula can be performed at a later stage when revision surgery is planned. After the first post-operative week, re-entering the abdomen is difficult and the patient may not have a peritoneal cavity. This patient appears to have a controlled fistula. It is therefore prudent to refrain from immediate surgery and manage her according to the above principles. Re-operating before a minimum of 3 months is fraught with risk of intestinal injury; therefore a period of 6 months is the best option here.

4   C – Wait 6 months and operate
Reversal of a Hartmann's procedure may be more difficult than the initial bowel resection because of the presence of dense adhesions and identification of the rectal stump. Therefore, it is suggested to wait for a period of 6 months before attempting a reversal as, by that time, the adhesions may be more conducive to surgery.

61 RECTAL BLEEDING

1 B – Anal fissure
Pain on defaecation can be due to an anal fissure, anal carcinoma or strangulated haemorrhoids. Haemorrhoids per se are not painful. Anal fissures are common in young adults and have an increased incidence following pregnancy.

2 F – Crohn's disease
This history is typical of inflammatory bowel disease. The most likely diagnosis here would be Crohn's disease in view of the weight loss and a palpable mass. These latter features are uncommon in ulcerative colitis.

3 A – Anal carcinoma
Anal carcinoma has a strong association with human papillomavirus (types 16, 18, 33) infection. The everted edge is characteristic of a neoplastic process and a carcinoma should be suspected. Bleeding is another common presentation of anal carcinoma.

62 POST-OPERATIVE PYREXIA

1 D – Pelvic abscess
The most likely diagnosis here is that of a pelvic abscess. This is the most common intra-abdominal infective complication following surgery for perforated appendicitis. Tenderness on rectal examination should also alert one to this complication.

2 H – Urinary tract infection
Urinary tract infection can be a cause of pyrexia in any post-operative patient from day 3 onwards. It should be considered in all patients who are catheterised for more than 5 days.

3 A – Anastomotic leak
Following any intestinal resection, especially those involving the large bowel, failure to progress in an 'uncomplicated' fashion (ie absence of pyrexia, tachycardia, oliguria, abdominal distension) should alert one to the possibility of an anastomotic leak.

4 G – Subphrenic abscess
The classic complication following repair of a perforated duodenal ulcer is a subphrenic collection. This should be suspected in a patient with a pyrexia, right upper quadrant signs or right basal collapse.

63 SCROTAL PAIN AND SWELLINGS

1 A – Epididymo-orchitis
The history here is characteristic of an acute epididymo-orchitis. The preceding urinary symptoms and raised WBC make the diagnosis most likely. The most common causative organisms are the Gram-negative bacilli. Thus therapy is most appropriately directed towards these.

2 C – Inguinoscrotal hernia
The presence of veins on the scrotal skin here is a red herring. Varicoceles do not cause large swellings in the hemiscrotum per se, but also disappear in the recumbent position. The inability to get above the swelling is a clinical sign of an inguinoscrotal hernia.

3 F – Testicular teratoma   ? *Ans - Seminoma (LDHT)*
Testicular cancer usually presents in the 20–40-year age group. It may be asymptomatic, but there is often a history of incidental trauma – the reason for this is unknown. Seminomas most commonly occur in 30–40-year-olds. In contrast, teratoma occurs in a younger age group (20–30 years). The α-fetoprotein produced by yolk-sac elements is raised in teratomas but not in seminomas. Trophoblastic cells secrete β-HCG and this may be present in either tumour.

4 H – Torsion hydatid of Morgagni
The differential diagnosis here is that of testicular torsion and torsion of a hydatid of Morgagni. The very localised tenderness and the presence of the bluish discoloration would make the latter the more likely diagnosis.

64 SUTURE MATERIAL

1   B – 3 '0' PDS

Numerous suture materials can be used for bowel anastomoses. The most popular materials are the absorbable ones: PDS (polydioxanone) and Vicryl. Non-absorbable materials can also be used, including Ethibond. The size of the suture would vary from 2'0' to 4'0'. Stapling techniques have become commonplace with the advantage of speed and a wider functional side-to-side anastomosis. There is no evidence that anastomotic leak rates are any higher between suturing and stapling.

2   G – 1 PDS

The abdominal wall can be closed through a variety of techniques: layered closure or mass closure. The latter is quicker and currently the most popular technique in the UK. The suture material may be absorbable or non-absorbable, loop or non-loop. However, it must be strong and heavy (usually a 1 PDS or 1 Nylon).

3   H – Stainless steel wire

Sternotomy wounds in adults are closed with stainless steel wires. However, sternotomy wounds in paediatric patients are closed with a heavy PDS suture.

4   D – 6 '0' Prolene

Arterial anastomoses are fashioned with prolene, an non-absorbable material, but gortex has also been used. For small calibre anastomoses fine material must be used, otherwise narrowing would occur.

5   E – 2 '0' Prolene

Prosthetic mesh techniques have become the accepted means for repairing incisional hernias. The aim is for the mesh to be secured in position and not migrate; therefore, a non-absorbable suture such as 2 '0' prolene is most appropriate.

65 DYSPHAGIA

1   A – Achalasia
Achalasia is a failure of relaxation at the lower end of the oesophagus because of loss of ganglia from the Auerbach's (myenteric) plexus. It affects females more than males (3 : 2) and is common during the third decade of life. There is progressive dysphagia to solids and liquids, chest pain and regurgitation of old food from the dilated oesophageal sac. Radiologically, achalasia is diagnosed by finding a dilated oesophagus with a tapering lower oesophageal segment, likened to a bird's beak, which fails to relax. There is no gastric air bubble because the dilated oesophagus never completely empties and, therefore, swallowed air cannot pass into the stomach. Chest X-ray shows air or fluid level behind the heart and the expanded oesophagus gives the appearance of a 'double right heart border'.

2   C – Oesophageal carcinoma
Carcinoma of the oesophagus is 1.5–3 times more common in men than in women. It is rare before the age of 40. Although the majority of tumours worldwide are squamous cell tumours, adenocarcinomas are the most common pathological type in the lower third, most resulting from Barrett's metaplasia. Dysphagia is the commonest presenting symptom. Other symptoms include: retrosternal discomfort, atypical chest pain from a secondary motility disorder, pulmonary symptoms or pneumonia caused by overspill and anaemia. Complications include tracheo-oesophageal fistula causing cough during eating, aorto-oesophageal fistula causing massive haematemesis (rare) and hoarseness of voice as a result of recurrent laryngeal nerve involvement (mainly in extensive middle-third tumours). Lymph node metastasis is common. Barium swallow and endoscopy are the mainstays of diagnosis.

3   F – Pharyngeal pouch
Pharyngeal pouch occurs more often in the elderly in whom they often have a long and symptom-free natural development. The patient presents with dysphagia and regurgitation of undigested foods (which has collected in the pouch), and subsequent weight loss. Pulmonary overspill is a problem and, on occasions, hoarseness and chest infection may be the only presenting symptoms. A mass low down in the anterior triangle of the neck may be felt and deep palpation over this may produce a squelching sound, caused by free fluid in the pouch.

4   B – Diffuse oesophageal spasm
Diffuse oesophageal spasm presents with intermittent dysphagia for solids and liquids and retrosternal chest pain. This condition may mimic a myocardial infarction as the pain radiates to the jaws or the inter-scapular region. The attacks may be associated with facial pallor and extreme sweating. The diagnosis of this condition has increased since the use of coronary angiography for the investigation of suspected anginal chest pain. Endoscopy is usually unremarkable and barium swallow may reveal the intense muscle contractions which may appear as a 'cock screw'. The 'nutcracker oesophagus' refers to the manometric finding of high-amplitude peristaltic contractions of long duration. The first line of treatment in a patient with diffuse oesophageal spasm is a thorough explanation of the cause of the pain and this itself may occasionally suffice.

66 ABDOMINAL PATHOLOGIES

1   B – Carcinoma of the rectum
Colonic malignancy is the second most common cause for cancer deaths in the UK. Predisposing factors include neoplastic polyps, ulcerative colitis, familial polyposis and a positive family history. Clinical presentation depends on the site: classically left-sided colonic carcinoma presents with obstructive symptoms, bleeding per rectum, altered bowel habit and tenesmus. In contrast, right-sided tumours usually present with symptoms of anaemia from occult bleeding. Sometimes the patient complains of pain in the right iliac fossa and abdominal examination may reveal a mass over this region. In both cases, a change in bowel habit is seen. These symptoms are not mutually exclusive and in many cases there is considerable overlap.

2   C – Crohn's disease
Crohn's disease is common in North America and Northern Europe. Unlike ulcerative colitis, Crohn's disease affects the whole of the GI tract (from mouth to anus). Risk factors include a strong positive family history; smoking increases the risk threefold. Acute Crohn's disease may mimic acute appendicitis. In chronic Crohn's disease, there is mild diarrhoea, extending over many months accompanied by intestinal colic; intermittent fever, secondary anaemia and weight loss. With progression of the disease, adhesions, trans-mural fissures, intra-abdominal abscesses and fistulas may develop.

3 H – Ruptured ectopic pregnancy

Ectopic pregnancy occurs in less than 1% of pregnancies. The typical history of ectopic pregnancy is one or two missed menstrual periods with other signs of pregnancy (mastalgia, morning sickness and increased urinary frequency). In ruptured ectopic pregnancy the abdominal pain is initially crampy, but subsequently becomes a more persistent and generalised lower abdominal pain. Irritation of the diaphragm leads to shoulder tip pain. There may be signs of hypotension and hypovolaemic shock. Internal examination may reveal guarding, rigidity and rebound tenderness. Frequently, altered blood may be seen in the cervix and movement of the cervix produces abdominal discomfort. In some instances a mass may be felt in one of the adnexae and the uterus is frequently soft and bulky. Ruptured ectopic pregnancy warrants immediate surgical intervention.

4 F – Mesenteric infarction

Although any of the three anterior abdominal aortic branches (coeliac, superior and the inferior mesenteric vessels) may occlude, it is the occlusion of the superior mesenteric artery (SMA) that is most commonly seen and causes mesenteric infarction. Despite the presence of collateral vessels in the SMA, an acute reduction in blood flow may not enable them to dilate sufficiently and rapidly enough. Occlusion may be due to a thrombus or an embolus. Causes of infarction include: atrial fibrillation, and more rarely, dissecting aneurysms and vasculitis. Clinical features include persistent, severe and generalised abdominal pain. Inflammatory markers may be elevated and arterial blood gases may reveal a metabolic acidosis. This condition is a surgical emergency, as the patient rapidly becomes toxic and may die from septic shock unless the infarcted bowel is removed.

67 ACUTE ABDOMINAL PAIN

1 D – Biliary colic

Biliary colic presents with pain in the RUQ/epigastric region usually (but not invariably) 2–3 hours after a fatty meal. The pain is sometimes associated with nausea and vomiting. There are no inflammatory signs, such as raised temperature or increased WCC, which may be present when the obstruction leads to acute cholecystitis.

2   J – Ruptured spleen
Rupture of the spleen is usually the result of a closed injury caused by direct external violence, typically by the steering wheel of a car or the handlebars of a bicycle. At all ages, splenic enlargement from malaria, infectious mononucleosis, vascular malformations and haematological malignancies all predispose the spleen to rupture following trivial trauma. Clinical features include signs of internal haemorrhage and pain referred to the left shoulder because of irritation of the diaphragm (Kehr's sign). Local signs include upper abdominal guarding, local bruising and abdominal distension.

3   G – Perforated peptic ulcer
Perforated peptic ulcer is common in patients who are on regular long-term NSAIDs. Perforation of a viscus causes sudden, severe pain which is usually appreciated in the area of the perforation – upper epigastric in the case of duodenal ulcer. There may be shoulder tip pain if the diaphragmatic peritoneum is inflamed. The patient may lie motionless and supine with shallow respiratory excursions. An erect chest X-ray reveals free gas under the diaphragm. Serum amylase may be mildly elevated (> 100 iu/ml) in some patients. Surgical intervention is required and the patient must be fully resuscitated before surgery with intravenous fluids, nasogastric tube, adequate analgesia and appropriate antibiotics. Surgery involves patching the perforation with greater omentum or performing a direct closure.

4   H – Ruptured abdominal aortic aneurysm
Risk factors for aortic aneurysm include: male sex, advancing age, hypertension, tobacco smoking, chronic obstructive airways disease (irrespective of tobacco smoking), infection of the vessel (eg salmonella), and occlusive arterial disease affecting the coronary, carotid and the limb arteries. A diagnosis of leaking or ruptured abdominal aortic aneurysm should be considered in the elderly with sudden onset of upper abdominal/periumbilical pain radiating to the back and associated with signs of progressive shock. Collapse is common and the patient is often pale and clammy with a low volume pulse. Acute pancreatitis is the other diagnosis to be considered. In ruptured aortic aneurysm, immediate surgical intervention is mandatory.

68 CHEST AND THORACIC WALL INJURIES

1   I – Tension pneumothorax

Tension pneumothorax occurs following penetrating injuries to the chest. This is a surgical emergency as it may result in cardiorespiratory arrest if the tension is not relieved immediately. With each inspiration air is drawn into the pleural space and has no route to escape (acting as a one-way valve). Patients present with respiratory distress, distended neck veins and deviation of the trachea to the opposite side. There is a shift of the mediastinum to the contralateral hemithorax. The immediate management is insertion of a large bore needle (cannula) into the second intercostal space in the mid-clavicular line on the affected side. Following this an intercostal chest drain must be inserted and connected to an underwater seal.

2   B – Diaphragmatic rupture

Diaphragmatic rupture occurs in high-speed blunt abdominal trauma against a closed glottis. Diaphragmatic rupture is more common on the left as the liver acts as a protective buffer on the right side. Bowel sounds may be heard in the chest. An X-ray may reveal bowel gas in the lung fields as the colon and stomach may herniate into the thorax. The surgical approach (trans-thoracic or trans-abdominal) depends on the stage of recognition and the presence of associated injuries. If detected early and with associated intra-abdominal injuries, a trans-abdominal approach is acceptable.

3   F – Perforated oesophagus

Spontaneous perforation of the oesophagus (Boerhaave's syndrome) is a result of severe barotrauma. The pressure in the oesophagus rapidly increases and the oesophagus perforates (tears) at its weakest point (lower third). The usually history is that of a patient experiencing severe chest or upper abdominal pain following a heavy meal or a bout of drinking (usually bingeing). Haematemesis may or may not be present. This condition may be misdiagnosed as a myocardial infarction or perforated peptic ulcer. Severe upper abdominal rigidity may be seen, even in the absence of peritoneal contamination.

4   A – Cardiac tamponade
Cardiac tamponade occurs following trauma, lung or breast carcinoma, pericarditis and myocardical infarction. The signs include: raised JVP, falling BP and muffled heart sounds (Beck's triad). In addition, with inspiration the JVP rises (Kussmaul's sign) with a fall in systolic blood pressure of more than 10 mmHg (pulsus paradoxus). Chest X-ray reveals a globular heart; the left heart border is convex or straight and the right cardiophrenic angle is < 90°.

69   SURGICAL INVESTIGATIONS

1   A – Abdominal CT scan
2   C – Barium enema (double contrast)
3   E – ERCP
4   E – ERCP
Hepatic hydatid disease characteristically results in complex cysts with septation and daughter cysts and is best seen on CT. Double contrast barium enema is the most precise method of demonstrating the presence and extent of uncomplicated diverticular disease. Colonoscopy carries a high risk of complication in patients with diverticular disease.

Endoscopic retrograde cholangiopancreatography (ERCP) defines ductal anatomical detail well, and may reveal the 'chain of lakes' of sclerosing cholangitis. Ultrasound may fail to show ductal dilatation or common duct stones. ERCP would provide a more definitive diagnosis and allow therapeutic manoeuvres for choledocholithiasis.

70   ABDOMINAL PAIN INVESTIGATIONS – DIAGNOSTIC

1   F – Erect chest X-ray
The first patient is most likely to have a perforated duodenal ulcer and an erect chest X-ray would be the best investigation.

2   I – Supine abdominal X-ray
The most likely diagnosis in the second patient would be a sigmoid volvulus and the supine X-ray would show an 'omega loop'.

3   F – Erect chest X-ray
The most likely diagnosis in the third patient is a perforated peptic ulcer and an erect chest X-ray would be most appropriate. Air is seen under the diaphragm in 90% of cases.

71 HERNIAS

1 B – Epigastric hernia
2 E – Obturator hernia
3 C – Gluteal hernia

Epigastric hernias are often painful and may be multiple. Treatment is by suturing the defect in the linea alba.

Obturator hernias may present in old women as a cause of medial thigh pain. Obturator hernias are often difficult to diagnose and may only be found at the time of surgery for small bowel obstruction.

72 NON-MALIGNANT CUTANEOUS LUMPS

1 E – Lupus vulgaris

Lupus vulgaris (Mycobacterium infection of the skin) usually occurs at 10–25 years of age. It appears as single or multiple cutaneous nodules (apple jelly-like) commonly over the face and neck. These lesions tend to heal in one area as it extends to another. The mucous membrane of the mouth and nose are sometimes affected, either primarily, or as an extension from the face. Infection of the nasal cavity may lead to the necrosis of the underlying cartilage. Oedema occurs if the fibrosis caused by the lupus obstructs the normal lymphatic drainage. Treatment is by anti-tuberculous chemotherapy.

2 G –Sebaceous cyst

Sebaceous cysts (epidermoid cyst) are intra-dermal lesions containing keratin and its breakdown products with a wall of stratified squamous keratinising epithelium. These cysts occur over the hairy areas of the body and may be inherited in an autosomal dominant fashion. Sebaceous cysts have a characteristic punctum, usually in the centre of the lesion, which blocks the sebaceous outflow. Treatment is by surgical excision. Since recurrence is common, complete removal of the cyst wall is essential.

3   H – Seborrhoeic keratosis
Seborrhoeic keratoses (basal cell papilloma, seborrhoeic wart) are benign tumours caused by the overgrowth of epidermal keratinocytes. They commonly occur after the age of 40. They are frequently pigmented and often develop as single or multiple, round or oval shaped slightly greasy lesions with a 'stuck on' appearance. Sometimes they occur in crops in sun-exposed areas (the trunk, face and arms) and are often characterised by a network of crypts. Multiple seborrhoeic keratosis may rarely be associated with an internal malignancy, eg colon carcinoma (Leser–Trelat sign).

4   B – Dermatofibroma
Dermatofibromas (fibrous histiocytoma, sclerosing haemangioma) are firm (woody), well defined, indolent, and single or multiple nodules usually found over the extremities. They are usually seen in the young or middle aged and are more common in women. They are freely mobile over the underlying tissues. Mild trauma or insect bites may trigger this and has led to the belief that they are not true tumours but the result of a tissue reaction. Histologically, some tumours are cellular, being composed largely of histiocytes while others are fibrous and composed of fibroblasts and collagen; yet others have a predominant angiomatous component. Treatment is by simple excision of the nodule.

73   CUTANEOUS MALIGNANCIES

1   H – Lentigo maligna
Of all malignant melanomas, lentigo maligna melanoma (Hutchinson's melanotic freckle) is the least malignant variety. It is more commonly seen in the elderly (over 60 years). It presents as an irregular brown patch commonly over the sun exposed parts (mainly cheeks and the dorsum of the hand). Malignant changes are recognised by the thickening and the development of a discrete tumour nodule. Histologically, there are islands of malignant melanocytic cells within the dermis and there is atrophy of the epidermis.

2 I – Nodular melanoma

Nodular melanoma is a most malignant type. It may occur over any part of the body, but it is commoner on the upper back (both sexes) and the lower legs of women. The lesions are overtly palpable, deeply pigmented, and usually convex in shape; they may bleed or ulcerate. The tumour has a smooth surface and an irregular outline but is sharply delineated from the surrounding skin. It has a poor prognosis with early lymphatic involvement. The management depends on the depth of invasion from its origin in the epidermis and the presence or absence of metastatic disease.

3 C – Basal cell carcinoma

Basal cell carcinoma, the most common cutaneous malignancy, commonly occurs in the sun-exposed areas of the elderly. They may be single or multiple. There is an increased incidence in smokers, in patients with xeroderma pigmentosa, and in previous radiotherapy scars. In the most common type of basal cell carcinoma (nodular or the nodulo-ulcerative type), the tumour usually commences as a small, waxy or pearly nodule with a clearly defined margin. The pearly appearance is more apparent on lightly stretched skin but may be covered with surface telangiectasia. As the tumour enlarges, central ulceration occurs, resulting in the characteristic rolled-out edge. Various modalities of treatment are advocated including surgical excision, fractionated radiotherapy, Mohs' micrographic surgery, cryosurgery, electro-dissection and curettage, topical chemotherapy (with 5-fluorouracil), CO_2 laser, intralesional interferon, and photodynamic therapy; the last three, however, remain largely experimental.

4 G – Keratoacanthoma

Keratoacanthoma is the 'self-healing' squamous cell carcinoma (SCC). It may be solitary or multiple, and is mostly seen in sun-exposed sites. It presents as a fleshy, elevated and nodular lesion with an irregular crater shape and a characteristic central hyperkeratotic core. The most significant histologic feature is its rapid growth. The short history and a rapid increase in size suggest keratoacanthoma rather than an SCC. In some cases keratoacanthomas undergo spontaneous resolution within 6 months of onset. If there is failure of resolution, complete surgical excision is the treatment of choice. Intralesional 5-fluorouracil is also useful in its management.

74 UPPER LIMB NERVE INJURIES

1   C – Injury to the upper cord of the brachial plexus
Upper brachial plexus or supraclavicular plexus lesion (C5, C6) occurs because of excessive depression of the shoulder or displacement of the head that opens out the angle between the shoulder and the neck (Erb-Duchenne paralysis). In neonates, it may occur following traction on the shoulder girdle during difficult labour or in breech delivery. In adults, it may occur as a result of a fall of weight on the shoulder or an RTA where the head is moved away from the shoulder. There is loss of shoulder abduction, elbow flexion and forearm supination. Consequently, the affected limb is internally rotated, extended at the elbow and pronated. There is sensory loss over the outer aspect of the arm and forearm.

2   E – Median nerve
In adults, the median nerve (C5–T1) is commonly injured near the wrist, although it can be injured anywhere along the arm or the forearm. Low lesions may be caused by lacerations in front of the wrist or by carpal dislocation. In children, supracondylar fractures of the humerus may lead to median nerve injury at the elbow. Median nerve injuries at the wrist cause sensory loss over the thumb, index, middle and occasionally ring finger (lateral half); motor loss includes all thenar muscles except adductor pollicis (supplied by ulnar nerve) and the lateral two lumbricals. If the injury is at the level of the elbow, there is paralysis of the pronators of the forearm and flexors of the wrist and fingers, with the exception of flexor carpi ulnaris and the medial part of flexor digitorum profundus.

3   H – Radial nerve
The radial nerve (C5–T1) is damaged at the mid-humerus level by fractures or pressure (prolonged tourniquet). Damage is seen in patients who fall asleep with the arm dangling over the back of a chair ('Saturday night palsy'). Radial nerve injury causes paralysis of the brachioradialis, the wrist extensors and extensor digitorum, leading to wrist-drop along with paralysis of extensors of the wrist, fingers and the thumb; there may be a small patch of sensory loss over the dorsum of the thumb and the first web space. In higher lesions, sensation is also lost on the dorsum of the forearm.

4   J – Ulnar nerve
The ulnar nerve (C8, T1) is an important motor nerve of the hand. Pressure (from a deep ganglion) or lacerations at the wrist may cause low lesions. Lesion of this nerve at the wrist produces hypothenar wasting and clawing of the hand as a result of the action of unopposed long flexors; there is loss of sensation over the little and ring fingers. Finger abduction is weak and the loss of thumb adduction makes pinch difficult. Consequently, paralysis of the adductor pollicis and the first palmar interosseous causes flexion of the thumb (due to flexor pollicis longus) – when the patient is asked to grasp a card between his thumb and index finger (Froment's sign).

75 AORTIC BYPASS GRAFTING

1   A – Aortobifemoral bypass
2   B – Axillobifemoral bypass
3   A – Aortobifemoral bypass
An aortobifemoral bypass graft has the highest patency rate of any bypass procedures to the femoral vessels.

An axillobifemoral bypass graft should only be considered in the very high-risk surgical patient who has critical ischaemia. It should not be performed in patients with claudication.

76 LOWER LIMB ISCHAEMIA

1   G – Percutaneous balloon angioplasty
Percutaneous balloon angioplasty is particularly suitable for localised stenoses and short occlusions. Lesions in the larger proximal vessels (above knee) are technically easier to treat, with fewer complications and better long-term results.

2   C – Femorodistal bypass
Femorodistal bypass using an autogenous vein graft is the treatment of choice in the second patient. Absence of contrast in the posterior tibial, anterior tibial and common peroneal arteries on angiography films must not be accepted as evidence of their occlusion.

3   H – Tissue plasminogen activator (TPA) infusion (intra-arterial)
Intra-arterial thrombolysis with TPA is the treatment of choice in the third patient in view of the short history (4 hours), angiographic findings and absence of neurological deficit.

4   F – Lifestyle changes only
The initial treatment of intermittent claudication is correction of risk factors, such as diabetes, hypertension, smoking and exercise. Younger non-smokers should have a thrombotic screen performed on presentation. Critical ischaemia is defined by rest-pain of at least 2 weeks' duration that requires regular adequate analgesia, or ulceration or gangrene of the foot or toes with an ankle pressure of < 50 mmHg or a toe pressure of < 30 mmHg.

5   B – Fasciotomy
The fifth patient has compartment syndrome. Urgent fasciotomy is indicated in order to save his right leg.

77   LOWER LIMB VENOUS DISEASE

1   B – Elevation, rest, NSAIDs and antibiotics
The woman with thrombosed varicose veins and cellulitis should be treated with elevation, rest, NSAIDs and antibiotics.

2   D – IV heparin
One should also suspect a deep-vein thrombosis in a patient with a swollen and tender leg post-operatively. It is best to perform some imaging (duplex Doppler study) before commencing treatment for this second scenario.

3   C – Emergency surgery
A patient with venous insufficiency and profuse bleeding from an ulcer should have emergency surgery to stop the bleeding.

78   CAROTID ARTERY DISEASE

1   B – Carotid Doppler
Thirty per cent of carotid bruits heard on auscultation are not because of carotid stenosis. The initial investigation that should be performed here is a Doppler ultrasound scan. This may be followed by digital subtraction angiography or magnetic resonance angiography (MRA), but many centres will rely on colour duplex Doppler alone if performed by an experienced operator.

2   C – CT scan
In cases where a persistent neurological deficit has occurred a CT scan must be carried out initially to exclude a space-occupying lesion.

SIN~

Answers

79 INVESTIGATION OF CAROTID ARTERY DISEASE

1 C – Duplex Doppler ultrasound of carotid arteries
Duplex Doppler ultrasound of the carotid arteries is the initial investigation of choice for carotid stenosis. It is the quickest and safest investigation for amaurosis fugax. Subsequently, carotid angiography (digital subtraction angiography) or MRA may be used to confirm the duplex findings.

2 B – CT scan of head
The 28-year-old with the dense stroke is most likely to have had an intracranial bleed necessitating a CT of the brain.

3 F – Transcranial Doppler ultrasound
Transcranial Doppler measures the flow in the middle cerebral artery and is thus useful in the intraoperative monitoring and investigation of post-endarterectomy neurological episodes. Duplex Doppler would also demonstrate patency of the carotid artery following endarterectomy. Near-infrared spectroscopy measures intracerebral blood flow but is not currently used for intraoperative monitoring.

80 VASCULAR TUMOURS

1 B – Chemodectoma
Chemodectomas originate from paraganglionic cells at the carotid bifurcation. If untreated, 5% metastasise within 10 years.

2 A – Angiosarcoma
Angiosarcomas usually develop in the extremities. Although they are radiosensitive and respond to chemotherapy, radical amputation is still advised.

3 E – Kaposi's sarcoma
A Kaposi's sarcoma is a haemangiosarcoma, treated with a combination of chemo- and radiotherapy.

4 D – Glomus jugulare tumour
A glomus jugulare tumour arises at the jugular bulb. Excision is associated with palsies of cranial nerves X, XI and XII. It should not be confused with a glomus tumour, which is the only true benign blood vessel tumour (cavernous haemangiomas are dilated blood spaces with thin walls, and port-wine stains/telangiectasias are capillary malformations). Most glomus tumours occur on the upper limbs, especially the digits.

81 LEG ULCERS

1 D – Postphlebitic
2 B – Diabetic
3 A – Arterial

Leg ulcers often have multiple aetiologies. The aetiology is usually apparent from taking a clear history and identifying the site of the ulcer. The most common causes of leg ulcers are venous, mixed, arterial, neuropathic, vasculitic (including rheumatoid arthritis) and neoplastic. Venous and postphlebitic ulcers tend to be situated in the gaiter area and have sloping edges.

Arterial ulcers have punched-out edges and often occur at pressure areas at the extremities, eg toes.

Diabetic ulcers often occur at the site of trauma or ill-fitting shoes. Neoplastic ulcers have raised, rolled or everted edges and may occur anywhere.

82 CAROTID ARTERY DISEASE

1 E – Right carotid endarterectomy
2 D – MRI head
3 E – Right carotid endarterectomy

Patients with carotid territory TIAs, amaurosis fugax or a stroke (with subsequent recovery), and a > 70% stenosis should be offered endarterectomy. The risks of the operation are less than the risk of suffering a disabling stroke, providing the operation is performed within 6 months of the stroke. Endarterectomy should carry a mortality of < 2%, and a 1–2% risk of stroke. It is normally too late to operate on completely occluded arteries. Patients with lesser degrees of stenosis should be given antiplatelet drug therapy.

A young patient with optic neuritis and foot drop should first have an MRI scan of the brain to look for demyelinating disease.

83 VARICOSE VEINS

1 D – Varicose vein surgery

Varicose veins must be dealt with surgically if they are suspected of causing an ulcerating lesion that is bleeding intermittently – this should be done promptly.

2 B – Elevation and NSAIDs

Episodes of thrombophlebitis are best treated by elevation, analgesics (NSAIDs are useful) and external elastic support.

3 C – IV heparin

On confirmation of a DVT, patients should be started on intravenous heparin as soon as possible. Intravenous heparin has been the mainstay of treatment; however, patients are frequently treated with low-molecular-weight heparins on an outpatient basis before starting warfarin therapy. Warfarin therapy aims to prevent the formation of clots; heparin aims to prevent their propagation and dispersal.

84 LOWER LIMB ISCHAEMIA

1 E – Surgical embolectomy

The first patient is likely to have had a mural thrombus post MI that has embolised to his leg. He may also have been in atrial fibrillation previously. As he has critical ischaemia, surgical embolectomy is indicated.

2 A – Angioplasty

Angioplasty is useful for short stenoses. This has better results for proximal stenosis above the inguinal ligament. For occluded vessels the procedure is now possible in specialist centres using cutting-balloon or subintimal angioplasty techniques.

3 D – Femoropopliteal bypass graft

A patient with rest pain has critical ischaemia and needs urgent intervention. A 10-cm stenosis is too long for a successful angioplasty. A good distal run-off would allow distal bypass grafting. The SFA is the commonest site for lower limb atherosclerosis because the vessel narrows as it passes through the adductor hiatus.

Answers

85 5-YEAR GRAFT PATENCY RATES

1   E – Reversed vein femoropopliteal graft
2   C – Femoral–femoral crossover graft
3   B – Axillofemoral graft
4   D – Femoropopliteal PTFE graft patency (below knee)
5   A – Aortobifemoral graft

Patency rates are related to the force and volume of the inflow and the run-off away from the graft. If the run-off is poor then blood that passes into the graft will be functionless; therefore, flow will be greatly reduced so leading to graft occlusion and failure. Synthetic grafts used below the inguinal ligament are vastly inferior to vein grafts.

86 LOWER LIMB ULCERATION

1   F – Pyoderma gangrenosum

Pyoderma gangrenosum is recurring nodulo-pustular ulceration that commonly affect the legs, abdomen and face. The ulcers are tender with a red-blue overhanging necrotic edge and they heal with cribriform scars. Pyoderma gangrenosum is associated with inflammatory bowel disease, acute leukaemia, polycythaemia rubra vera, autoimmune hepatitis, Wegener's granulomatosis and myeloma.

2   J – Venous ulcer

Venous ulcers may develop spontaneously or following a minor injury. Risk factors include past history of varicose veins and deep-venous thrombosis (DVT); all causes of varicose veins or DVT may therefore predispose to venous ulceration. Venous incompetence leads to a high venous pressure which causes pericapillary fibrin deposition, white cell activation and increased production of free radicals. All these factors contribute to skin breakdown, causing ulceration. These ulcers usually lie proximal to the medial or lateral malleolus, although they may extend to the ankle or dorsum of the foot. Lipodermatosclerosis frequently accompanies long-standing venous incompetence. Increased exudate leads to venous eczema, excoriation of the surrounding skin, itch and worsening of the ulcer.

Answers

3   E – Neuropathic ulcer
Neuropathic ulcers can result from peripheral sensory neuropathy secondary to diabetes mellitus. The other causes for altered sensory neuropathy, leading to neuropathic ulcers include: spinal cord injuries, spina bifida, tabes dorsalis, syringomyelia, alcohol abuse and leprosy. Neuropathic ulcers are common at the sites of pressure or repeated trauma. The usual sites in the lower limb are the head of the metatarsals, interdigital clefts, heel (calcaneum) and the lateral malleolus. In diabetic patients, the arterial blood pressure index (ABPI) may be falsely elevated, because of calcification of the vessel walls and medial sclerosis, even in those with major vessel disease. Neurological assessment of the foot and toes may reveal altered sensation including proprioception and two-point discrimination, reduced vibration sense and absent ankle jerks.

4   G – Sickle cell disease
Sickle cell disease is hereditary haemolytic anaemia occurring mainly among those of Afro-Caribbean origin. The haemoglobin 'S' molecule crystallises during reduced blood oxygen tension causing vascular occlusion. Depending on the affected vessel, patients may have bone or joint pain, priapism, neurological abnormalities, skin ulcers. Ulceration is due to occlusion of the cutaneous microcirculation, leading to ischaemia and skin breakdown. In dark-skinned individuals, there may be a non-specific increase in melanin pigmentation around the ulcer which, if over the ankle region, may be confused with haemosiderin discoloration around a venous ulcer.

87   RENAL TRANSPLANT

1   C – Chronic rejection
2   A – Acute rejection
3   B – Blood group mismatch
4   D – Hyperacute rejection

Hyperacute rejection occurs immediately, as a result of a reaction from pre-existing antibodies to the transplanted tissue, eg ABO blood type mismatch.

Acute rejection occurs as a result of HLA type mismatch, and is controlled by matching donor and recipient HLA types and with immunosuppressive drugs.

The humoral immune system is responsible for chronic rejection, which can take months or years to occur.

88 PAEDIATRIC INVESTIGATIONS

1 B – A 'double-bubble sign' on plain AXR
Persistent bile-stained vomiting (if the atresia is distal to the second part where the common bile duct enters the duodenum) in a newborn infant may indicate a diagnosis of duodenal atresia. The typical radiological feature is the 'double-bubble' seen on plain AXR (an air-filled dilated stomach and first part of duodenum, creating two discrete air shadows).

2 H – Intramural gas on plain AXR
A premature baby presenting with bile-stained vomiting and rectal bleeding is at high risk of suffering from necrotising enterocolitis. The typical radiological feature of this condition is gas within the bowel wall on plain AXR. It may be associated with gas in the portal system and/or free air in the abdomen when the disease progresses to intestinal perforation.

3 C – A 'target' lesion on abdominal ultrasound
An 8-month-old infant with colicky abdominal pain and rectal bleeding is likely to have intussusception, which may be diagnosed on abdominal ultrasound by the presence of a 'target lesion' or by gastrografin enema. The 'target' lesion represents the layers of the bowel, one invaginated inside the other, seen in transverse section.

4 A – A 'cone' on contrast enema
Hirschsprung's disease typically presents in the first few days of life with abdominal distension, bile-stained vomiting and failure to pass meconium. The diagnosis can easily be made by the presence of a cone between collapsed distal (usually rectum) and proximal dilated bowel on a contrast enema. The cone represents the transition zone between normal proximal ganglionated bowel and distal aganglionic bowel. Confirmation of Hirschsprung's disease, however, can only be made on histological biopsy.

89 PAEDIATRIC CONDITIONS

1   A – Intussusception
A sausage-shaped mass may be seen in intussusception or pyloric stenosis. However, bilious vomiting is not a feature of pyloric stenosis. Rectal bleeding with the production of 'redcurrant jelly' stools is seen in intussusception.

2   C – Pyloric stenosis
The patient in question has typical features of pyloric stenosis.

3   B – Meckel's diverticulum
Meckel's diverticulum may give rise to rectal bleeding as 5% of cases have ectopic gastric mucosa.

90 NEONATAL SURGICAL DIAGNOSES

1   D – Hirschsprung's disease
Hirschsprung's disease usually presents in the neonatal period with a history of delayed passage of meconium, abdominal distension and bile-stained vomiting. The infant may be shocked with impending enterocolitis. Hirschsprung's disease is more common in children with Down's syndrome (trisomy 21). It can be differentiated postnatally from duodenal atresia in which there is passage of meconium, even in complete atresia.

2   B – Exomphalos
Both gastroschisis and exomphalos are frequently diagnosed antenatally. In exomphalos, the liver is frequently outside the abdomen and the herniated organs are covered by an identifiable membrane.

3   F – Mid-gut volvulus
Bile-stained vomiting in a previously well infant should raise the suspicion of a mid-gut volvulus.

4   H – Oesophageal atresia
A baby with oesophageal atresia is frequently born to a mother with polyhydramnios. At birth the infant is unable to swallow even saliva, which froths through the mouth and nose.

5   I – Tracheo-oesophageal fistula

Oesophageal atresia can occur with or without a tracheo-oesophageal fistula, which itself can occur in isolation. When an infant feeds, there may be aspiration of milk through the fistula into the lungs. Occasionally, the infant may be several months old before the diagnosis is made.

91 PAEDIATRIC NEWBORN GASTROINTESTINAL DISORDERS

1   B – Duodenal atresia
2   D – Intussusception
3   C – Hirschsprung's disease

A child with a scaphoid abdomen and bilious vomiting should be suspected of having duodenal atresia. Symptoms usually occur in the first few hours of life. The diagnosis may be made by injecting 30 ml of air via a nasogastric tube and taking a radiograph. This is not to be confused with the persistent vomiting of hypertrophic pyloric stenosis, which is not bile stained and presents at 6 weeks.

A child with an abdominal mass, distension, passing meconium for 3 days and now passing blood, should be suspected of having an intussusception. It is only late in the disease that bleeding per rectum becomes a feature, suggesting mucosal necrosis.

Meconium ileus tends to present with a distended abdomen and bilious vomiting with no passage of meconium. The rectum is characteristically empty. Distal small bowel obstruction, secondary to abnormally bulky viscid meconium is seen in 1 : 15 000 newborns. Ninety per cent of these infants will have cystic fibrosis.

Hirschsprung's disease is the most common cause of intestinal obstruction in a newborn and affects 1 : 5000 children. Typically, there is delay in passing meconium beyond the first 24 hours of life with abdominal distension and bilious vomiting. Patients with Hirschsprung's disease may present after the neonatal period with chronic constipation or partial large bowel obstruction.

92 GASTROINTESTINAL DISORDERS IN NEONATES

1   E – Intussusception
Intussusception is caused by invagination of a segment of bowel into its adjoining lower segment. It is more common in boys and usually occurs under 1 year. Intussusception is associated with haemophilia, Henoch–Schonlein purpura, haemangiomas and GI lymphomas. Clinical features include severe colicky abdominal pain (causing intermittent inconsolable cries with the child drawing up the legs) and vomiting. Between attacks, the infant may appear in good health. The infant may pass 'redcurrant jelly' stools and a sausage-shaped mass is palpable on abdominal examination. Rectal examination may reveal blood.

2   G – Meconium ileus
Meconium ileus is seen in 1 in 15 000 newborns. This is due to distal small bowel obstruction secondary to abnormally bulky and viscid meconium. Ninety per cent of these infants will have cystic fibrosis and the viscid meconium is the result of deficient intestinal secretions. The condition presents during the very early days of life with gross abdominal distension and bilious vomiting. X-ray of the abdomen shows distended coils of bowel and a typical mottled 'ground glass appearance'. Fluid levels are scarce, as the meconium is viscid.

3   I – Necrotising enterocolitis
Necrotising enterocolitis is more common in premature infants. Terminal ileum, caecum and the distal colon are the commonly affected sites. The abdomen is distended and tense, and the infant passes blood and mucus per rectum. Mesenteric ischaemia causes bacterial invasion of the mucosa leading to sepsis. Erythema of the anterior abdominal wall suggests full-thickness necrosis of the bowel with peritonitis. X-rays of the abdomen shows distended loops of intestine and gas bubbles may be seen in the bowel wall.

4   B – Hirschsprung's disease
Hirschsprung's disease is an absence of ganglion cells in the neural plexus of the intestinal wall. It is more common in males. The delayed passage of meconium together with distension of the abdomen following feeds and bilious vomiting are the usual clinical features. Plain abdominal X-ray may demonstrate dilated loops of bowel with fluid levels. Barium enema demonstrates a 'conical appearance' in the affected part as a result of the dilated ganglionic proximal colon and the distal aganglionic bowel failing to distend.

93 DISORDERS OF THE BONE

1   G – Osteopetrosis
Osteopetrosis is an autosomal recessive condition. The patient, usually a young adult, may present with symptoms of anaemia (tiredness) or thrombocytopenia (recurrent throat and chest infections) because of decreased marrow space. Deafness and optic atrophy can result from compression of the cranial nerves. Blood investigations may reveal a leukoerythroblastic picture. The bones are very dense and brittle, and X-ray reveals a lack of differentiation between the cortex and the medulla described as 'marble bone'.

2   F – Ostegenesis imperfecta
Osteogenesis imperfecta (brittle bone disease) is defective osteoid formation due to the congenital inability to produce adequate intercellular substances, such as osteoid, collagen and dentine. In addition, there is a failure of maturation of collagen in all the connective tissues. Some typical clinical features of this condition include: a broad skull, blue sclera, premature deafness, scoliosis, ligament laxity, coxa vara and knock knees. X-rays may reveal translucent bones, multiple fractures particularly of the long bones, wormian bones (irregular patches of ossification), and a trefoil pelvis.

3   J – Scurvy
Scurvy (vitamin C deficiency) causes a failure of collagen synthesis and osteoid formation. The patient, usually a child or an infant, may present with swelling and tenderness near the large joints. There may be bleeding from the gums as they are spongy. Spontaneous bleeding may lead to subperiosteal haematoma and the child remains still (pseudoparalysis) as a result of subperiosteal bleeding. X-rays shows generalised bone rarefaction. The metaphysis may be deformed or fractured. Vitamin C in the form of ascorbic acid should be given in doses of 1 gm/day and the child should be encouraged to eat fresh fruit and vegetables.

4   I – Rickets

Rickets is the childhood form of osteomalacia. Because of vitamin D deficiency osteoid fails to ossify. Symptoms start from about the age of 1 year. The child may present with tetany or convulsions. The child is small for age and there is a history of failure to thrive. Bony deformities include: bowing of the femur and tibia, deformity of the skull (craniotabes), deformity of the chest wall with thickening of the costochondral junction (ricketty rosary), and a transverse sulcus in the chest caused by the pull of the diaphragm (Harrison's sulcus). The characteristic X-ray change is an increase in the depth and width of the epiphysis and the adjacent metaphysis has a 'cupped' appearance; these changes are most noticeable in the wrist.

94   PELVIC FRACTURE

1   B – Rotationally unstable, vertically stable pelvic fracture
Rotationally unstable, vertically stable pelvic fractures include open-book fractures (pubic diastasis > 2.5 cm) and lateral compression fractures.

2   B – Rotationally unstable, vertically stable pelvic fracture
Rotationally unstable, vertically stable pelvic fractures include open-book fractures (pubic diastasis >2.5 cm) and lateral compression fractures.

3   C – Rotationally unstable, vertically unstable pelvic fracture
Rotationally and vertically unstable pelvic fractures usually result from vertical shear injuries.

4   A – Rotationally and vertically stable
Stable pelvic fractures include fractures not displacing the pelvic ring (such as avulsion fractures and isolated fractures of the iliac wing or pubic ramus) or minimally displaced fractures of the pelvic ring.

5   A – Rotationally and vertically stable
Stable pelvic fractures include fractures not displacing the pelvic ring (such as avulsion fractures and isolated fractures of the iliac wing or pubic ramus) or minimally displaced fractures of the pelvic ring.

95 PERIPHERAL NERVE ANATOMY

1 A – Axillary
The axillary nerve passes just below the capsule of the shoulder joint and is damaged here in about 5% of shoulder dislocations. The nerve gives off the upper lateral cutaneous nerve of the arm, and also motor branches to the deltoid and teres minor muscles. The multipennate fibres of the deltoid muscle contract isometrically when carrying weights in the hand. The strap/unipennate anterior and posterior slips of the muscle are used for flexion and extension and, when contracting together, take over from the supraspinatus muscle to abduct the arm beyond the first 15°.

2 H – Thoracodorsal
The thoracodorsal nerve is most vulnerable to damage during axillary surgery, when the arm is laterally rotated and abducted, because it bows into the axilla from the posterior wall. Paralysis of the latissimus dorsi muscle is detected clinically if the patient is unable to fold the arm behind the back and reach up to the opposite scapula. The intercostobrachial (sensory) nerve is also vulnerable and, occasionally, has to be sacrificed.

3 G – Suprascapular
The suprascapular nerve, which is motor to the supraspinatus and infraspinatus muscles, may be damaged by sudden tightening of a car seat-belt (upper trunk injuries of the brachial plexus and clavicular fractures may also occur). Paralysis of both muscles weakens the rotator cuff, destabilising the shoulder joint. In addition, the supraspinatus abducts the arm from 0° to 15°, and the infraspinatus is a powerful lateral rotator of the humerus. Since the teres minor muscle is unaffected (axillary nerve), some lateral rotation is preserved after suprascapular nerve damage.

4 F – Radial
Mid-shaft fractures of the humerus can damage the radial nerve in the spiral groove. The branches to the triceps are given off before the nerve enters the groove and so the muscle remains functional. All other extensors are paralysed, resulting in wrist drop. Although the cutaneous branches no longer conduct, compensatory overlap by adjacent nerves restricts the paraesthesia/anaesthesia to the dorsal skin over the first interosseous muscle. The brachioradialis reflex is mediated by the radial nerve and is thus lost. The triceps reflex remains intact for reasons explained above.

5   B – Long thoracic
The long thoracic nerve usually escapes damage during axillary surgery because it is bound to the serratus anterior muscle by overlying fascia on the medial wall, posterior to the mid-axillary line. When the nerve is injured, however, part or all of the serratus anterior muscle is paralysed, resulting in a 'winged scapula'. There is loss of protraction and weakness of rotation of the scapula (the latter movement is, however, preserved by the action of the intact trapezius muscle – spinal accessory nerve).

96   SHOULDER PAIN

1   D – Supraspinatus rupture
A complete tear of the supraspinatus tendon may occur after a long period of chronic tendonitis. Active abduction is impossible and attempting it produces a characteristic shrug; however, passive abduction is full and once the arm has been lifted to above a right angle the patient can keep it raised using the deltoid (abduction paradox).

2   E – Supraspinatus tendonitis
Supraspinatus tendonitis usually occurs in patients < 40 years of age who develop shoulder pain after vigorous/strenuous exercise. On active abduction the scapulohumeral rhythm is disturbed and pain is aggravated as the arm traverses an arc between 60 and 120°.

97 LOW BACK PAIN

1 G – Spondylolisthesis
Spondylolisthesis commonly presents in the teenage years with pain and hamstring tightness. This is not the same as a limited straight leg raising where the 'strain' is on the sciatic nerve.

2 D – Muscle strain
Muscle strains are the most common cause of low back pain in fit young adults, particularly if there has been some 'unaccustomed' exercise. A slipped disc is more likely to be associated with radiation of the pain and symptoms of nerve root irritation.

3 E – Osteoporotic collapse
Many 88-year-olds have osteoporosis and a simple fall can cause an osteoporotic fracture with collapse. As the patient is improving, a more sinister explanation is unlikely.

4 A – Discitis
In children who refuse to walk, a septic arthritis or osteomyelitis affecting the lower limbs must first be excluded; only then may a diagnosis of discitis be considered.

5 C – Metastatic disease
Although the gentleman here is relatively young, the history of progressive pain radiating to the buttocks and cauda equina symptoms must raise the concern of a metastatic lesion.

98 COMPLICATIONS OF HIP SURGERY

1 D – Urinary retention, male
2 A – Death
3 E – Wound infection without prophylaxis
4 B – Deep-vein thrombosis (DVT), no prophylaxis
5 C – Pulmonary embolus, no prophylaxis
Prophylaxis has had a marked impact on the reduction of deep wound infections and thrombotic complications. The risk of deep wound infection has dropped from 1–5% to < 1% and the risk of a DVT from 60% to 15%. The risk of a PE in a patient on low-molecular-weight heparin is now 1–5%.

99 KNEE INJURIES

1 F – Tibial plateau fracture
2 E – Patellar fracture
3 C – Injury to the medial meniscus
4 A – Anterior cruciate rupture
5 D – Medial ligament rupture

A valgus force to the knee produced by a car bumper is likely to result in bony damage (a tibial plateau fracture); a similarly directed force during a game of football is more likely to lead to rupture of the medial collateral ligament. Complete rupture of this ligament would lead to gross instability on weight-bearing at the time of injury. As the joint is disrupted, no discrete effusion is seen, although the area may be swollen and bruised.

Swelling due to a medial meniscal injury usually takes some hours to become apparent. However, an anterior cruciate ligament rupture with the classical 'pop' produces a rapid haemarthrosis.

100 HEAD INJURY

1 A – Basal skull fracture
Fractures of the skull vault may be linear, comminuted or depressed. Bruising over the mastoid process (retro-auricular bruising – 'Battle's sign') and periorbital haematoma (raccoon eyes) are classic signs of basal skull fractures. Middle fossa fractures present with rhinorrhoea/otorrhoea (blood mixed CSF and it does not clot), haemotympanum, ossicular disruption, and VII and/or VIII cranial nerve palsies.

2 E – Extradural haematoma
Acute extradural haematoma should be suspected after a head injury where the patient has a fluctuating level of consciousness (though not invariably). The patient may briefly lose consciousness, but soon recovers (lucid interval). An acute extradural haematoma is usually associated with trauma and seen in young adults. Extradural bleeds are commonly the result of fractured temporal or parietal bones and injury to the middle meningeal artery or vein. Blood loss (and haematoma formation), with lateralising signs, including an ipsilateral dilated pupil and contralateral hemiparesis, develop. This eventually leads to a bilateral fixed pupils and coma, culminating in respiratory arrest.

3 H – Subaponeurotic haematoma

In contrast to localised scalp haematomas, subaponeurotic haematomas are diffuse, arising in the space between the galea and the pericranium. They usually occur a few days after a head injury. They present as a large, diffuse and fluctuant swelling underneath the scalp, extending from the frontal region to the occiput. They may be associated with swollen eyelids. These haematomas do not need aspiration as they gradually resolve over a number of weeks.

4 J – Subdural haematoma

About 20% of subdural haematomas are bilateral. Although most subdural haematomas are secondary to trauma, spontaneous subdural haematomas can occur in elderly patients with cerebral atrophy. Alcoholics, epileptics, and patients on anticoagulants are particularly susceptible. In chronic subdural haematomas, patients may not become symptomatic for many days or even weeks after head injury (trivial in many cases). They may then present with headache, fluctuating levels of consciousness (not usually seen in acute subdural), failing intellect and hemiparesis.

101 JOINT AND BACK PAIN

1 A – Ankylosing spondylitis

Ankylosing spondylitis, predominantly seen in the young, affects more men than women (6 : 1). The patient presents with morning stiffness, backache, progressive loss of spinal movements leading to kyphosis, and hyperextension of the neck (question mark posture). Occasionally, patients may present with unstable fractures after minor trauma. X-rays show a 'bamboo spine' with squaring of the vertebrae. Blood test reveals raised ESR, normochromic anaemia and positive HLA-B27 antigen.

2 B – Intervertebral disc herniation

Lumbar disc herniation (prolapse) commonly occurs in fit young adults usually when lifting heavy weight or while straining. A sudden acute pain is felt in the lower back, and it may be accompanied by shooting pain radiating to the buttock or down the leg along the appropriate nerve roots. Examination reveals paravertebral muscle spasm, leading often to a 'spinal tilt' and a global reduction in spinal movements. Straight leg raise (SLR) is often restricted to < 50° and reproduces the radicular symptoms.

3   G – Reiter's syndrome

Reiter's syndrome (sexually acquired reactive arthritis) is a triad of urethritis, conjunctivitis and seronegative arthritis. The patient is usually young; the disease affects large joints and causes oligo- or mono-arthritis. Other features include iritis, keratoderma blenorrhagica (brown, aseptic abscesses on soles and palms), circinate balanitis (painless serpiginous penile rash), plantar fasciitis and Achilles tendonitis. Management includes NSAIDs, rest, and splintage of the affected joint.

4   J – Spondylolisthesis

Spondylolisthesis is the slipping forward of one vertebra in relation to another. Isthmic spondylolisthesis is one type (of five) and appears to be a form of repetitive stress fracture; the incidence is much higher in teenage gymnasts and other athletes. It commonly occurs between the ages of 7 and 10. The signs and symptoms include low backache, hamstring spasm, fifth lumbar nerve root pain, and disturbance in the sagittal profile of the spine with an acute kyphosis. In some cases, neurological symptoms may affect the legs. On examination, there may be a step in the line of the spinous processes; straight leg raising may be reduced because of hamstring spasm.

102 LOWER LIMB PATHOLOGIES

1   C – Compartment syndrome

Compartment syndrome may develop after trauma (accident) or surgery. It results from an increase in pressure within an osseofacial compartment, leading to compromise of the microcirculation and nerve and muscle damage. The microcirculation is compromised if compartment pressures rise above 30–40 mmHg (or the difference between the diastolic pressure and the compartment pressure is < 30 mmHg). With increasing compartment pressures, the capillary perfusion is inadequate to meet the metabolic demands of the intracompartmental tissues. The patient complains of unremitting pain that is not relieved by morphine. Loss of sensation in the early stages precedes motor loss – loss of peripheral pulses is usually a late, but sinister sign. Irreversible injury occurs with pressures as low as 30 mmHg for 6–8 hours.

2   D – Deep-vein thrombosis
Hospitalisation and immobility increase the incidence of deep-vein thrombosis. The other risk factors include: increasing age, pregnancy, oral contraceptive pill, surgery especially orthopaedic or pelvic, malignancy, past history of DVT and thrombophilia. In addition, any factor contributing to venous stasis, vein wall damage and increased coagulation of blood (known as Virchow's triad) predisposes to formation of a clot. Clinical features of DVT include redness, swelling, pain, calf tenderness, dilated superficial veins (sometimes), and low-grade pyrexia. These signs and symptoms usually develop after 7–10 days post-operatively.

3   G – Milroy's syndrome
The peak age of onset of Milroy's disease (primary lymphoedema; lymphoedema praecox) is 10–30 years, and it has a clear genetic predisposition in some patients. This condition is the result of congenital absence of the lymphatics. It is more common in females and is seen shortly after menarche. It is more likely to be unilateral. The swelling usually develops around the ankle and the dorsum of the foot which soon spreads proximally extending up to the knee. Occasionally, patients develop numerous vesicles in the skin which may leak clear lymph or, occasionally chyle. The swelling is worse during the day and decreases at night.

4   H – Ruptured Achilles tendon
Rupture of the Achilles tendon is common in patients over the age of 40, probably because the tendon is frayed. It usually occurs when the patient is involved in unaccustomed activities, such as running or jumping; sudden contraction of the calf muscle is resisted by the body weight and the tendon ruptures. The patient feels as if he or she has been struck just above the heel and is usually unable to continue with the involved activity. Soon after the tear, a gap can be felt about 5 cm above the insertion of the tendon. The patient is unable to tiptoe and plantar flexion of the ankle (or foot) is weak or lost. Simmond's test is positive (reduced plantar flexion of the ankle on squeezing the calf muscle). The management is either conservative (using plaster casts) or surgical (with the foot plantar flexed, the cut ends are approximated and held in place using non-absorbable sutures 2/0 nylon). Following this, the ankle and the foot are immobilised in a below-knee plaster cast in equinus position for 6–8 weeks.

103 LOWER LIMB NERVE INJURY

1   C – Lateral cutaneous nerve of thigh
Lateral cutaneous nerve of the thigh compression (meralgia paraesthetica) may cause pain and paraesthesia over the upper, lateral aspect of the thigh. Sensation may also be decreased over this area. It may be seen in pregnancy or any condition which causes a pressure on this nerve within the pelvis (eg tumours). The symptoms are usually self-limiting.

2   A – Common peroneal nerve
Common peroneal nerve (lateral popliteal nerve; L4–S2) injury is common following fibular neck fractures since the nerve winds down the neck and is relatively superficial at this point. This nerve gives motor supply to the dorsiflexor and eversion muscles of the ankle and toes. Its sensory branches supply the anterior and lateral aspect of the leg and whole of the dorsum of the foot and toes, except the skin between the great and the second toe (supplied by deep peroneal nerve). Injuries result in foot drop and the patient is unable to dorsiflex or evert the foot. Sensory loss is over the anterior and lateral aspect of the leg, and dorsum of the foot and toes.

3   B – Femoral nerve
The femoral nerve (L2–4) may be injured by a gunshot wound, traction during surgery, injury to the femoral triangle or by massive haematoma within the thigh, and in patients with diabetes mellitus and lumbar spondylosis. There is weakness of the quadriceps muscle causing weak knee extension. Patients find that the knee gives way on walking and have difficulty climbing stairs. There is numbness over the anterior thigh and medial aspect of the leg. The knee jerk is depressed.

4   H – Sciatic nerve
Sciatic nerve (L4–S3) injury is common following traumatic dislocations of the hip (posterior dislocation), total hip replacement and other traction injuries to the nerve. A complete lesion will affect all the muscles below the knee, leading to loss of knee flexion, foot drop and an inability to walk. Patients drag their feet behind them and are often unable to stand for prolonged periods. Calf muscle wasting is a long-term complication. There is loss of sensation below the knee on the lateral side (medial side is supplied by the saphenous nerve). The knee jerk is normal but the ankle jerk is lost.

104 BONE AND CONNECTIVE TISSUE TUMOURS

1 I – Osteosarcoma

Osteosarcoma, the most frequently encountered malignant lesion of bone, is characterised by the direct formation of bone or osteoid tissue by a sarcomatous stroma. It typically affects the knee and the proximal humerus in the metaphyseal region. The incidence is highest in the 10–25-years age group. Secondary osteosarcoma, however, may arise in the bones of the elderly affected by Paget's disease (in approximately 10% of patients affected for > 10 years) or after irradiation. The characteristic symptoms of pain, local tenderness, a soft tissue mass and a decreased function may be present for variable periods of time. On examination, the affected part is swollen and the overlying skin may be shiny and warm. The lump is tender and has irregular edges. The ESR may be raised. X-ray shows bone destruction and new bone formation, often with marked periosteal elevation ('Sunray spiculation' and 'Codman's triangle', respectively). Surgical excision is the treatment of choice.

2 B – Ewing's sarcoma

Ewing's sarcoma is a malignant tumour arising from the vascular endothelium of the bone marrow. The tumour is common in the 10–20-years age group and occurs in the diaphysis of the long bones. Clinical features include pain and swelling; the lump is warm and tender, with ill-defined edges. The ESR may be elevated, thus spuriously suggesting an inflammatory or infective cause such as osteomyelitis, although osteomyelitis usually affects the metaphyseal region in children. X-rays often show a large soft-tissue mass with concentric layers of new bone formation – known as 'onion-peel' sign. Treatment includes chemotherapy and surgical excision.

3 F – Osteochondroma

Osteochondroma (cartilage-capped exostosis) is the most common benign tumour of the bone. The usual site for the tumour is the metaphysis of the long bones. The lesion may be single or multiple (hereditary multiple exostoses). The usual history is of a lump that is discovered accidentally. The lump is bony hard and non-tender. X-ray reveals a well-defined swelling; however, the swelling looks smaller than it feels because of the invisible cartilaginous cap.

4   G – Osteoclastoma

Osteoclastoma (giant cell tumour) is an uncommon, aggressive, locally destructive lesion seen in the metaphyseo-epiphyseal region of long bones. It frequently occurs in young adults 20–40 years of age and is more common in women. The principal sites are the distal femur, proximal tibia, proximal fibula, distal radius and proximal humerus. On examination, a vague swelling is felt at the end of long bones and the neighbouring joint is often inflamed. Although < 5% of these tumours metastasise, the lesions are extremely destructive, sometimes locally resulting in pathological fractures (approximately 10% of cases) as seen in this patient. X-ray shows thinning of the cortex giving it an expanded appearance – the characteristic 'soap bubble' appearance. Radiotherapy is the treatment of choice.

105 SHOULDER JOINT PATHOLOGIES

1   G – Painful arc syndrome

In painful arc syndrome (chronic supraspinatus tendonitis; impingement syndrome), there is pain on abduction 60–120° (middle 1/3 of the arc), but the extremes of movements are painless. The underlying pathology is the swelling of the tendon, and the pain is produced when it impinges on the undersurface of the acromial process during the mid-phase of abduction. Repeating the movement with the arm in full external rotation throughout may be much easier and relatively painless; this is virtually pathognomonic of painful arc syndrome.

2   H – Rotator cuff tear

Rotator cuff is a sheet of conjoint tendons (subscapularis, supraspinatus, infraspinatus and teres minor) closely applied to the shoulder capsule and inserting into the greater tuberosity of the humerus. The differing clinical pictures stem from three basic pathological processes – degeneration, trauma and vascular lesion. The supraspinatus tendon is liable to injury when it contracts against firm resistance; this may occur when lifting a weight, or when the patient uses his or her arm to save themselves from falling. This is much more likely if the cuff is already degenerate. The clinical presentation reflects the loss of tendon function with weakness, a drop arm sign (characteristic hunching of the affected shoulder) and even inability to lift the arm. There is often relentless night pain. On local palpation, pain is felt at the shoulder-tip and upper arm and there is tenderness under the acromion.

3   C – Calcific tendonitis
Calcific tendonitis is a common disorder of unknown aetiology which results in an acutely painful shoulder joint. Frequently, there is no history of trauma. Calcium becomes deposited within the supraspinatus tendon and this may be part of a degenerative process. Clinical features include sudden onset of pain with no apparent precipitating cause. Pain in usually felt over the anterolateral aspect of the shoulder and is worse with overhead activities. On examination, the shoulder is tender anterolaterally, with some restriction of both active and passive movements. External rotation, however, is possible (this feature differentiates the condition from frozen shoulder). X-ray reveals calcific deposits within the supraspinatus tendon, inferior to the acromion and medial to the tuberosity of the humerus.

4   D – Dislocated shoulder
Shoulder dislocation is common after trauma. Anterior dislocation is the commonest type (in contrast to posterior dislocation in the hip joint). Shoulder dislocation may be associated with injury to the axillary nerve which causes loss of sensation over the upper outer aspect of the deltoid region ('badge' area). The round contour of the shoulder is lost because of the absence of the head of the humerus within the glenoid fossa – the head of humerus may be felt in the deltopectoral groove (in anterior dislocation). Even in clinically obvious dislocations, an X-ray should be performed to rule out an associated fracture.

106 SPINAL PATHOLOGY

1   A – Acute disc prolapse
2   D – TB of the spine
Pain on hip extension represents a positive femoral stretch (L2, 3, 4). Only 5% of disc prolapses occur above L4–5. An acute disc prolapse will cause a scoliosis as a result of a muscle spasm.

Scheuermann's disease is of unknown cause, affecting 1% of the population and often associated with kyphosis. There is avascular necrosis of the ring apophyses and disc herniation through the endplate. It may be associated with excessive mechanical stress or endocrine abnormalities.

TB of the spine should always be suspected in patients from the Asian subcontinent. Note that the incidence of TB is increasing in the UK.

107 NERVE DAMAGE

1   B – Neurapraxia of the common peroneal nerve
2   C – Neurapraxia of the median nerve
3   F – Neurotmesis of the medial nerve
4   A – Horner's syndrome
5   H – Sciatic nerve injury

The peroneal nerve is very susceptible to pressure, and thus may result in a neurapraxia. Following a supracondylar fracture of a child's humerus, a neurapraxia of the median nerve is the most common neurological lesion but damage to the ulnar nerve is also not uncommon.

If a surgical procedure is complicated by nerve injury, a transection (neurotmesis) must be considered – especially if the nerve has not been visualised.

A flail upper limb suggests a brachial plexus lesion, which might well be associated with Horner's syndrome if the sympathetic chain is involved.

During a hip replacement, two forms of nerve injury are well documented: direct damage to the sciatic nerve at the level of the hip joint (more common); and pressure on the peroneal nerve at the neck of the fibula. During a posterior approach to the hip, the sciatic nerve is in particular danger.

108 HAEMORRHAGIC SHOCK

1   D – Blood loss of 0.75 litre
2   C – Blood loss of 2.5 litres
3   B – Blood loss of 1.7 litres
4   C – Blood loss of 2.5 litres
5   E – Blood loss of 1 litre

The effects of blood loss can be monitored in terms of physiology, ie pulse rate/blood pressure/pulse pressure/respiratory rate/urine output/CNS or mental status. Shock is graded I–IV depending on the amount of blood loss, and each grade is associated with certain physiological changes. Class I shock occurs when up to 15% of the blood volume is lost (up to 750 ml in a 70-kg adult); class II between 15 and 30% (750–1500 ml); class III between 30 and 40% (1500–2000 ml), class IV > 40% (2000 ml). The percentages are best remembered as the scoring system in a tennis match.

ORGANISMS

1 F – *Streptococcus pneumoniae*
Ludwig's angina is bilateral infection of the submandibular, sublingual and submental spaces – usually arising from dental sepsis. Streptococcal infection spreads in deep cervical and pharyngeal fascial planes. It may cause airway obstruction.

2 G – None of the above
Vincent's angina is due to the symbiotic action of fusiform bacteria and the spirochaete *Borrelia vincentii*. It is a pharyngeal infection with ulcerative gingivitis.

3 A – *Clostridium difficile*
After broad-spectrum antibiotic therapy, infection with *Clostridium difficile* may lead to pseudomembranous colitis

110 HEPATITIS B

1 C – Positive HBeAg in serum
2 D – Raised titre of anti-HBs antibody
3 D – Raised titre of anti-HBs antibody
4 A – HBsAg
The hepatitis B virus consists of an outer surface coat (HBsAg), and an inner core particle (HBcAg and HBeAg). Inside the core particle is the HBV DNA and DNA polymerase. The whole virus is called the Dane particle.

In acute infection, HBsAg is found in the blood and usually disappears after 3 months, at which point anti-HBsAg appears indicating immunity. HBeAg will also be seen early, and also disappears by 3 months, after which anti-HbeAg antibodies will be seen. In the 10% of patients who do not recover from the acute hepatitis infection, there is progression to chronic infection and the HBeAg and HBsAg will continue to be seen in the blood. This indicates continuing infection with the virus. If anti-HBe antibodies are present, the patient has seroconverted and his/her infectivity is lower. HBeAg represents replication of the virus and high infectivity. HBsAg represents a carrier status, if present for more than 6 months from onset of infection.

111 SKIN CONDITIONS

1   C – Necrotising fasciitis
Necrotising fasciitis is caused either by streptococcal infection or, more commonly, by mixed aerobic and anaerobic bacteria. It may occur in leg ulcers in patients with vascular insufficiency (and usually diabetes), as well as the perineum and scrotum (Fournier's gangrene). The patient is pyrexial and ill and the affected part becomes anaesthetic and gangrenous. The treatment is debridement of all necrotic tissue and antibiotics (penicillin based).

2   E – Pyogenic granuloma
A pyogenic granuloma is a haemangioma, which commonly occurs on the lips and fingers. This should not be confused with pyoderma gangrenosum, which is an ulcerated nodule or pustule with a tender, blue necrotic edge associated with inflammatory bowel disease, myeloproliferative disorders and inflammatory arthritides.

112 RENAL TRACT CALCULI

1   B – Extracorporeal shock wave lithotripsy (ESWL)
Stones measuring 2 cm in diameter, that lie within the kidney, are usually treated with ESWL. Percutaneous nephrolithotomy (PCNL) is used for a stone bulk > 2 cm (or > 1 cm in the lower pole calyx). ESWL can be used afterwards to residual fragments (called Steinstrasse, which have the appearance of a stone street in the ureter). Stones in the lower pole calyx have poor clearance rates and thus PCNL is the preferred option.

2   C – Nephrectomy
A staghorn calculus in a functional kidney is treated with PCNL followed by ESWL to remove residual fragments. However, in a patient with a 15% split function, the most appropriate treatment would be nephrectomy if the split function is < 15%.

3   E – Percutaneous nephrostomy
Obstructed infected kidneys need immediate drainage by percutaneous nephrostomy (from above).

Insertion of a ureteric stent (from below) is useful for preventing a stone causing a PUJ obstruction, for the prophylaxis of stones > 1 cm prior to more definitive treatment and to keep luminal patency after accidental or planned ureteric opening.

113 BENIGN PROSTATIC HYPERPLASIA

1   D – Retropubic (open) prostatectomy
2   F – TURP
3   F – TURP
The morbidity in patients with very large prostates (> 100 g) is less if open retropubic prostatectomy is performed rather than a transurethral resection of the prostate (TURP), as this reduces operation time and avoids excessive fluid absorption during prolonged surgery. Finasteride is a useful treatment in men with large (> 40 g) prostates. It also reduces prostatic bleeding.

One must always warn a patient undergoing TURP of the risk of retrograde ejaculation following the operation.

Catheterisation is not indicated in simple chronic urinary retention unless renal function is impaired.

114 TESTICULAR TUMOURS

1   E – Radiotherapy
2   E – Radiotherapy
3   F – Retroperitoneal lymph node dissection
The present treatment of stage I seminoma is radical orchidectomy and prophylactic radiotherapy to the retroperitoneal nodes, although trials are under way comparing adjuvant radiotherapy with carboplatin (adjuvant chemotherapy). More advanced seminomas should be treated with chemotherapy also. Intratubular germ cell neoplasia inevitably develops into cancer; therefore, a prophylactic radiotherapy dose of 20 Gy is given to the remaining testis after sperm banking has been offered. The treatment of residual nodes following chemotherapy and normalisation of tumour markers is retroperitoneal lymph node dissection.

Teratomas are much less radiosensitive and should be treated by orchidectomy and platinum-based combination chemotherapy.

115 TRANSITIONAL CELL CARCINOMA

1   H – Transurethral resection of bladder tumour
2   F – Nephroureterectomy
3   D – M-VAC chemotherapy

The treatment (in most cases) of a bladder tumour is a transurethral resection (TURBT) of the polypoid part of the tumour and a biopsy to stage muscle invasion. If it is found to be stage T_2–T_{4a}, one should perform cystectomy ± radiotherapy, plus chemotherapy if preferred.

The standard treatment of a transitional-cell carcinoma in either the kidney or ureter is a nephroureterectomy, as these tumours are often multifocal and surveillance of a ureteric stump is difficult. A cystectomy is contraindicated if enlarged pelvic lymph nodes are detected preoperatively.

116 IMAGING

1   G – Spiral CT scan

A non-contrast spiral CT with thin cuts will detect 'all' calculi. This imaging modality may be used when an IVU or ultrasound are contraindicated or impractical.

2   B – DMSA scan

Staghorn calculi require DMSA imaging to ascertain the split function of the kidneys, as DMSA is secreted by the kidney.

3   C – DTPA scan

DTPA scans are used to show which kidney is obstructed, as it is filtered by the glomerulus. MAG-3 is filtered and secreted, and is now the most commonly used isotope in imaging departments.

PUJ obstruction has a trimodal distribution: antenatal, teenagers (when they start drinking alcohol) and the elderly. A diuresis in a patient with a PUJ obstruction worsens the pain and should arouse suspicion of this condition.

117 SCROTAL SWELLINGS

1   H – Teratoma of testis
Ninety per cent of testicular neoplasms are germ cell in origin and the majority are malignant. Teratomas (seen in the 20–30-years age group) and seminomas (seen in the 30–40-years age group) are the commonest tumours. Others include: Sertoli cell tumours (causing feminising symptoms such as gynaecomastia) and Leydig cell tumours (causing sexual precocity). Approximately 10% of malignancies are found in undescended testes, even after orchidopexy. Most men present with a painless swelling, although 10% may present with an acutely painful testis. The usual presentation is a sensation of heaviness in the testis and the groin. A history of trauma is usually given in history. Testicular sensation is lost early. A small hydrocele may be present and the spermatic cord may be thickened from malignant infiltration. Trans-scrotal biopsies should never be performed and the initial management is orchidectomy.

2   I – Torsion of testis
Testicular torsion is common in children. Symptoms include sudden agonising pain in the groin and lower abdomen associated with vomiting. Torsion of the fully descended testis may be difficult to diagnose. A high-lying testis with thickening of the tender twisted cord is observed. Elevation of the testis worsens the pain (in contrast to epididymo-orchitis where elevation relieves the pain). However, these clinical signs are relatively non-specific and surgical exploration is mandatory if the diagnosis is suspected.

3   J – Varicocele
A varicocele is the varicose dilatation of the veins draining the testis. It is common in tropical countries and usually seen in tall, thin men with a pendulous scrotum. Varicocele is generally asymptomatic but at times may cause a vague and dragging discomfort. The scrotum on the affected side hangs lower than the other side. The cough impulse may be present (hence a differential for an inguino-scrotal hernia). When the patient stands the varicocele feels like a 'bag of worms'. On lying down, the swelling disappears as the veins empty. In long-standing cases, the affected testis is smaller because of atrophy. Varicoceles are associated with infertility. The sudden appearance of a varicocele in a middle-aged man should always raise the suspicion of retroperitoneal disease.

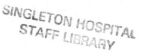

4   F – Primary hydrocele
Primary hydrocele is mostly seen in the middle aged. The common presenting complaint is a scrotal swelling. On examination, a cough impulse is absent, the swelling is dull to percussion and it is clinically possible to 'get above' it (thus distinguishing it from an inguino-scrotal hernia). The fluid of the hydrocele surrounds the body of the testis, making the testis impalpable. A hydrocele is fluctuant and trans-illuminates.

118 RENAL PRESENTATIONS

1   G – Renal calculi
Patients with renal calculi present with sudden severe flank or abdominal pain which may radiate to the scrotum or labia and/or into the ipsilateral costovertebral angle. The patient is restless and inconsolable (unlike in acute appendicitis and perforated viscera where he or she lies still). Urinalysis usually shows red blood cells. White blood cells may be seen if there is an associated infection. The development of calculi may be the result of altered metabolism and excretion of calcium, uric acid, cystine or oxalate. The calculi usually consist of the above elements either on their own or in combination. Investigations for suspected renal calculi include: plain radiography kidneys and upper bladder (KUB), IVU, ultrasound or a CT urogram (CTU). Calcium oxalate calculi make up about 90% of the stones. Since they are radio-opaque, they are visible in plain radiographs. Uric acid stones are virtually radiolucent.

2   A – Acute renal failure
The aetiology of acute renal failure could be classified into pre-renal (decreased renal perfusion due to haemorrhage, dehydration, burns, sepsis, etc), renal (nephrotoxic drugs, such as NSAIDs and angiotensin-converting enzyme inhibitors (ACE inhibitors)) and post-renal (ureteric and lower urinary tract obstruction) causes. This patient has developed acute renal failure secondary to obstruction because of renal calculi (only one kidney is present). It is essential to exclude obstruction as the cause for acute renal failure, particularly in patients with a solitary kidney. Obstruction needs to be relieved either surgically (neprostomy/extracorporeal shock wave lithotripsy) or radiologically (percutaneous) depending on the level and type of calculus and the patient's general health.

Answers

3   C – Focal segmental glomerulosclerosis
Focal segmental glomerulosclerosis is a recognised complication of renal transplantation. It has a higher incidence in intravenous drug abusers and in patients with HIV infection or AIDS. The condition presents with proteinuria, hypoalbuminaemia, oedema and hypercholesterolaemia. Biopsy of the kidney reveals focal glomerular deposits of IgM. More than 50% of the patients progress to chronic renal failure.

4   D – Gram-negative sepsis
This patient has developed Gram-negative sepsis as a result of instrumentation of the renal tract. The common organisms include *Escherichia coli* and bacteroides. Prophylaxis with an antibiotic such as gentamicin is usually recommended before surgery or instrumentation of the renal tract. Immediate management of Gram-negative sepsis entails antibiotics, oxygen and intravenous fluids.

119 RENAL TRACT PATHOLOGIES

1   A – Adenocarcinoma of the kidney
Adenocarcinoma of the kidney (hypernephroma; Grawitz's tumour) affects more males than females (2 : 1) and is more prevalent in patients over 40 years of age. Risk factors include smoking, genetic factors, a high intake of fat, oil and milk, and exposure to toxins, such as lead, cadmium, asbestos and petroleum products. Clinical features include: a dragging discomfort in the loin and a triad of haematuria (with occasional clot colic), flank pain (in 35–40%) and palpable abdominal mass (in 25–45%). In men, a rapidly developing varicocele (most often on the left) is a characteristic sign. This is because the left testicular vein drains into the left renal vein, whereas the right testicular vein drains directly into the inferior vena cava. The patient may also manifest symptoms of hypertension, erythrocytosis and hypercalcaemia.

2   E – Nephroblastoma

Nephroblastoma (Wilms' tumour) is a malignant mixed tumour seen in infancy. The tumours are usually solitary, soft, lobulated and are tan or grey in colour. The infant may present with pyrexia, haematuria (blood in the nappy), failure to thrive, and a non-tender abdominal (flank) mass. This mass does not cross the midline which distinguishes it from neuroblastoma (which usually crosses the midline), and is more nodular and irregular. Investigations include: blood count, biochemical profile, ultrasound scan (to confirm the mass and to also to view the other kidney), intravenous urogram (to give anatomical detail and an indication of renal function) and renogram. It is usually treated by total nephrectomy or partial nephrectomy (in children with bilateral disease) followed by radiotherapy.

3   H – Renal tuberculosis

Renal tuberculosis commonly occurs in the 20–40-years age group; it is more common in males than females (2 : 1) and the right kidney is affected more than the left. The symptoms are an increase in the urinary frequency (both during the day and night), painful micturition, renal pain and haematuria. Constitutional symptoms are weight loss and a slight evening rise in temperature. Chemotherapy (pyrazinamide, isoniazid, rifampicin) forms the basis of management of genitourinary tuberculosis. The anti-tuberculous drugs have high urinary excretion rates.

4   J – Transitional cell carcinoma of the bladder

Transitional cell carcinoma of the bladder usually occurs over the age of 50 and is more common in men. The aetiology of this condition includes cigarette smoking (more than 20 cigarettes/day has 2–6 times risk of developing bladder cancer), working in the aniline dye and rubber industry (because of excretion of β-naphthyl-amine in the urine), schistosomiasis infestation of the bladder and long-term catheterisation in paraplegic patients. Patients may present with painless haematuria, dysuria, frequency and urgency of micturition. Investigations include urine microscopy and culture (to rule out any infection) and cystoscopy. Endoscopic resection of the mass followed by a 4–6 week course of radiotherapy to the bladder and the pelvic side walls is useful in treating most tumours. Combination regimens of cisplatin, methotrexate and vinblastine (and adriamycin in some cases) are useful in the treatment of metastatic disease.

Answers

120 ACID–BASE BALANCE/STATUS

1 C – Pulmonary embolus
Pulmonary embolus (small or medium sized) usually produces a lowered P_{CO_2} because of increased respiratory rate.

2 A – Acute renal failure

3 D – Pyloric stenosis
Vomiting due to pyloric stenosis causes volume depletion and loss of H^+. The obstruction between the stomach and the duodenum also results in a decreased loss of HCO_3^-. A resultant metabolic alkalosis may occur if duodenal secretion continues and renal excretion of HCO_3^- is insufficient to correct for the plasma rise in HCO_3^-.

A flail chest occurs when a segment of the chest wall has no bony continuity with the rest of the thoracic cage. This usually results from trauma associated with multiple rib fractures. Underlying lung injury and restricted chest wall movement will contribute to the patient's hypoxia.

121 ACID–BASE BALANCE

1 D – Respiratory acidosis
Patients who suffer from chronic obstructive pulmonary disease (COPD) usually have a respiratory acidosis with a compensatory metabolic alkalosis. In cases where there is an infective exacerbation, respiratory acidosis becomes the predominant feature with marked CO_2 retention.

2 A – Metabolic acidosis
A serum amylase level of four times the normal value is pathognomic of pancreatitis. Patients with severe acute pancreatitis will usually be acidotic from a number of causes: hypovolaemic shock, acute renal failure and lactic acidosis.

3 E – Respiratory alkalosis
The third case is indicative of a pulmonary embolism (PE). The first indication of a PE is dyspnoea. The patient will be hyperventilating, so producing a respiratory alkalosis. Following a lobectomy, the blood gas analysis should not be grossly altered and the pH should be normal.

122 ACID–BASE BALANCE

		pH	Paco$_2$	HCO$_3^-$
1	A –	7.20	3.1	11
2	C –	7.56	3.0	30
3	B –	7.42	6.1	35

Intestinal obstruction would lead to loss of fluid from the intravascular space and produce third-space loss. The presence of peritonitis and a grossly elevated WBC strongly suggest the presence of infarcted bowel. All these factors would produce a metabolic acidosis.

The history in the second case is suggestive of pulmonary emboli. Pulmonary emboli may occur at any stage after surgery, but most frequently after 5 days, and should be suspected in all cases of dyspnoea (earliest sign). The ensuing hyperventilation would reduce Pco$_2$, shifting the Henderson–Hasselbach equation to the right (reducing H$^+$), causing a respiratory alkalosis.

Patient 3 may not be taking deep enough breaths due to pain from his laparotomy, which would be exacerbated by COPD from his smoking. He will therefore have a respiratory acidosis due to retained carbon dioxide. Note there is a compensatory rise in the serum bicarbonate level.

Normal values:

pH	7.35–7.45
Pao$_2$	>10.6 kPa
Paco$_2$	4.7–6.0 kPa
HCO$_3^-$	24–30 mmol/l

123 AUDIT

1 **D – Strategic**
2 **A – Criterion**

Audit is the systematic critical analysis of the quality of medical care, including the procedures used for diagnosis and treatment, the use of resources, resulting outcome and quality of life for the patient.

Audit may be subdivided into: medical audit (assessment of patient treatment by doctors) and clinical audit (assessment of patient treatment by all healthcare professionals).

INDEX

Note to reader: Entries are indexed by theme number, not by page number.

Index

Index

Index